CHOLESTEROL DOWN

BY JANET BOND BRILL

Cholesterol Down

Blood Pressure Down

Intermittent Fasting for Dummies

Prevent a Second Heart Attack

CHOLESTEROL DOWN

Ten **Simple Steps** to **Lower Your** Cholesterol in Four Weeks—**Without** Prescription Drugs

JANET BOND BRILL, PHD, RDN, FAND

Foreword by Jennifer H. Mieres, MD, FACC, FAHA

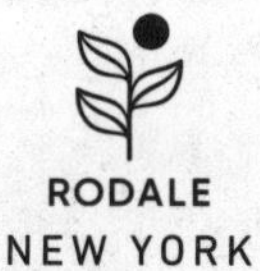

This book is not intended as a replacement for qualified, professional medical care. It is not intended to diagnose, prevent, treat, or cure any disease. Individuals with high cholesterol and/or those at risk for cardiovascular disease should first consult with their personal physician for medical clearance before making any of the dietary and lifestyle changes recommended in the Cholesterol Down Plan. The Cholesterol Down Plan should not be substituted for a physician-prescribed statin drug without the express permission of your personal physician. Statins have been scientifically proven to lower the risk of death from cardiovascular disease, whereas the Cholesterol Down Plan has not yet been shown to prevent heart disease or heart attacks. Several of the steps outlined may produce adverse reactions in some people and could potentially interact with over-the-counter and prescription medications. While every effort has been made to provide accurate and up-to-date information, this document cannot be guaranteed to be free of factual error. Consult your physician regarding applicability of any information provided in this book for your medical condition. The recipes are not intended for individuals prescribed special diets by their physician. Both the author and the publisher take no responsibility for any consequences that may arise from following the advice set forth within these pages.

Rodale Books
An imprint of Random House
A division of Penguin Random House LLC
1745 Broadway, New York, NY 10019
rodalebooks.com | randomhousebooks.com

LIBRARY OF CONGRESS CATALOGING-IN-PUBLICATION DATA
Names: Brill, Janet Bond author | Mieres, Jennifer H. writer of foreword
Title: Cholesterol down / Janet Bond Brill, PhD, RDN, FAND;
foreword by Jennifer H. Mieres, MD, FACC, FAHA.
Description: Revised edition. | New York, NY: Rodale, [2026] |
Previously published under title: Cholesterol down: ten simple
steps to lower your cholesterol in four weeks, without prescription drugs. |
Includes bibliographical references and index.
Identifiers: LCCN 2026005363 (print) | LCCN 2026005364 (ebook) |
ISBN 9780593980491 trade paperback | ISBN 9780307494467 ebook
Subjects: LCSH: Hypercholesteremia—Popular works | Hypercholesteremia—
Diet therapy—Popular works | Low-cholesterol diet—Popular works
Classification: LCC RC632.H83 B75 2026 (print) | LCC RC632.H83 (ebook)
LC record available at https://lccn.loc.gov/2026005363
LC ebook record available at https://lccn.loc.gov/2026005364

Originally published in different form in the United States by Harmony, an imprint of Random House, a division of Penguin Random House LLC, in 2006.

Printed in the United States of America

1st Printing

BOOK TEAM: Production editor: Dennis Ambrose • Managing editor: Allison Fox • Production manager: Richard Elman • Copy editor: Martin Schneider • Proofreaders: Andrea Gordon, Caryl Schwartz

Rx art: Recoonde/Adobe Stock

Book design by Lorie Pagnozzi

The authorized representative in the EU for product safety and compliance is Penguin Random House Ireland, Morrison Chambers, 32 Nassau Street, Dublin D02 YH68, Ireland. https://eu-contact.penguin.ie

This book is dedicated to my father, Rudy Bond, who died of a massive heart attack in 1982. Perhaps it was my father's untimely death from cardiovascular disease that ultimately inspired me to follow my career path in nutrition and wellness. I only hope that I can prevent others from suffering his same fate.

I also dedicate this book to my beloved husband, Sam, who has always supported me in all ways that have truly mattered: in my education, with our children, and in life. You are the ideal husband for me, for no other could have played your role in such a perfect way. Thank you, and I love you.

And to my children, Rachel, Mia, and Jason, who are simply my everything.

CONTENTS

FOREWORD

By Jennifer H. Mieres, MD, FACC, FAHA

Despite tremendous advances in the management and treatment of cardiovascular disease, it remains the leading killer of American men and women. This is at least in part due to unhealthy lifestyle choices, particularly when it comes to food and exercise.

Clinical research over the last several decades has provided overwhelming evidence that lifestyle and dietary factors influence risk of coronary heart disease (CHD)—both favorably and unfavorably. Specifically, the Lifestyle Heart Trial published in *JAMA* in 1998 was the first scientific study to demonstrate the powerful, positive impact of lifestyle changes such as diet, exercise, stress reduction, and smoking cessation on coronary heart disease.[1] Further data from both the Framingham Study and Multiple Risk Factor Intervention Trial (MRFIT) demonstrated that approximately 85 percent of controllable risk for premature coronary artery disease is the result of one or more major factors: elevated total cholesterol, high levels of LDL cholesterol, diabetes, smoking, advancing age, and a family history of premature heart disease.[2] The 2019 ACC/AHA Guideline on the Primary Prevention of Cardiovascular Disease AHA also emphasizes a comprehensive approach to cardiovascular health through sustainable lifestyle changes rather than short-term modifications.[3] The recommendations for adults include consuming a healthy diet that emphasizes the intake of vegetables, fruits, nuts, whole grains, lean vegetable or animal protein, and fish, as well as minimizing the intake of trans fats, red meat, processed red meats, refined carbohydrates, and sweetened beverages.

Creating lasting habits that support overall cardiovascular health and making the right changes in your food choices and lifestyle can significantly lower your risk of heart disease. On the other hand, living with excess body weight, consuming too much saturated fat, and having high cholesterol are three leading factors that contribute to the progression of atherosclerosis, which is the process of fatty cholesterol-filled plaque accumulating in the lining of the arteries. In particular, elevated levels of cholesterol have been directly linked to plaque buildup in the arteries that supply nutrients to the heart and brain, making high cholesterol a potent risk factor for all cardiovascular diseases, including heart attack and stroke. Data from the landmark Framingham Study and the Multiple Risk Factor Intervention Trial Research Group have established beyond a shadow of a doubt that LDL cholesterol is a significant contributor when it comes to plaque buildup in the arteries and the development of atherosclerotic cardiovascular disease (ASCVD). By taking simple measures to lower your LDL level, you can reduce your risk for heart disease and stroke—maybe even save your life.

In 2002 the National Cholesterol Education Program, an initiative of the federal government, published the Adult Treatment Panel III (ATP III), which clearly states that significantly reducing LDL cholesterol can halt the progression of atherosclerosis, or plaque buildup in the arteries, to prevent deaths from heart disease and stroke. The guidelines given by ATP III provide the scientific rationale as well as appropriate treatment recommendations for clinical cholesterol management, including both dietary changes and statin therapy, depending on the patient's category of risk.

The 1994 landmark Scandinavian Simvastatin Survival Study (4S), a trial of cholesterol lowering in 4,444 patients with coronary heart disease, clearly demonstrated the positive impact of simvastatin (a lipid-lowering statin drug) on reducing deaths from heart disease. According to this study, a mean reduction of cholesterol by 25 percent with the use of a statin was associated with as much as a 46 percent reduction in deaths and heart attacks from coronary heart disease.[4] The 2012 publication from the Cholesterol Treatment Trialists' (CTT) Collaboration highlighted the findings of a meta-analysis which analyzed data from twenty-seven studies, which included over 134,000 patients to study the effects of lowering LDL cholesterol with statin therapy. They found that over a 5-year period, for every 38 mg/dL reduction in LDL cholesterol through the use of statins, there was as much as a 21 percent reduction in cardiovascular events including death from heart disease.[5]

There is no question that the introduction of lipid-lowering medications, specifically statins, has significantly increased our treatment strategies for hypercholesterolemia (elevated levels of the soft, waxy fat cholesterol in the blood) and has clearly resulted in fewer deaths from all cardiovascular diseases. The current AHA prevention guidelines recommend statin therapy as first-line treatment for preventing ASCVD in patients who have elevated LDL cholesterol levels (≥190 mg/dL), those with diabetes mellitus, those who are between forty and seventy-five years of age, and those determined to have a sufficient ASCVD risk after consulting with a clinician.

However, many people remain fearful of the side effects of statins, are averse to the idea of taking prescription medications, or are unable to get their LDL cholesterol to the recommended level on drugs alone. Recent studies have demonstrated that combining specific foods (nuts, plant protein, viscous fibers, plant sterols) can reduce LDL-C by as much as 15 percent when combined with a healthy diet and provides similar outcomes as low-dose statin therapy.[6,7] According to the American Heart Association's "Life Essential 8," which describes the key steps for supporting cardiovascular health, a heart-healthy lifestyle that includes attention to diet and exercise can lower the risk of heart disease by as much as 80 percent.[8] Managing your lipids remains the cornerstone of addressing ASCVD, and there is a large and growing number of non-statin therapies available to manage elevated cholesterol levels.

For people who are statin hesitant and interested in a non-statin therapy, Dr. Brill's Cholesterol Down Plan provides an effective strategy to begin the process of cholesterol-lowering as a trial before using prescription drugs. In *Cholesterol Down,* Dr. Brill provides a practical, accessible approach for the reduction of LDL cholesterol levels without prescription drugs. Dr. Brill's plan is highly effective, and in addition to the scientific evidence to support her recommendations, the testimonials of her patients' success lend substantial credence to her approach. In cases where changes in diet and lifestyle may not be sufficient in lowering LDL cholesterol to recommended levels, lipid-lowering therapy (e.g., statins) may be prescribed as adjunct treatment.

On a personal note, one of my close friends came to me as a patient after learning she had an elevated total cholesterol level of 228 and LDL of 138 and triglyceride levels of 155.

Joanne's story was classic. She had a family history of elevated cholesterol (both mother and father took statins for elevated cholesterol levels), a family history of heart disease, and as she approached menopause from the age of forty-four to her current age of forty-six, she began to notice a yearly increase in her cholesterol levels. She was reluctant to start statin therapy and wanted to try changes in diet and exercise instead.

After reviewing her daily diet and routine, we both agreed that her diet and sedentary lifestyle were far from being heart healthy. She was ten pounds overweight, exercising at most twice a week, and put little effort into eating a balanced, low-fat diet. We agreed on a trial of lifestyle and diet modifications with a focus on the following six steps of

Dr. Brill's Cholesterol Down Plan: (1) Thirty minutes of exercise at least five days a week; (2) oatmeal; (3) apples; (4) beans; (5) almonds; and (6) six Metamucil capsules. In addition, I encouraged her to include more fruits and vegetables in her daily diet.

After four weeks on the plan, she had lost about six pounds and reduced her cholesterol levels to: total cholesterol of 213 (down from 228) and LDL of 117 (down 21 points from 138). HDL (good cholesterol) increased from 79 to 84. She is now determined to try all ten steps of Dr. Brill's Cholesterol Down Plan.

Like Dr. Brill, I believe it is of great importance that we be proactive and take ownership of our bodies and our heart health. The simple, consistent, and inexpensive lifestyle therapy outlined in her Cholesterol Down Plan could be the most important investment you make in your future health.

—Jennifer H. Mieres, MD, FACC, FAHA,
professor and associate dean, Donald and Barbara Zucker School
of Medicine at Hofstra/Northwell, and co-author of
Heart Smarter for Women: Six Weeks to a Healthier Heart

PREFACE

Heart disease continues its reign as America's most relentless killer, claiming more lives of both men and women than any other condition in the United States. Yet beneath this sobering reality lies a remarkable story of progress. According to the American Heart Association, the death rate from cardiovascular diseases has plummeted by half between 1924 and 2024—a transformation that translates into millions of lives extended and improved annually. This statistic isn't merely impressive; it represents one of medicine's greatest triumphs—a victory won through science, awareness, and individual action.

This dramatic shift didn't happen by chance. The introduction of revolutionary treatments like coronary stents, the awakening of public consciousness to heart-healthy living, the steady decline in smoking rates, and the development of potent LDL-lowering medications have all contributed to this quiet revolution in cardiovascular health. Each advancement, from sophisticated surgical techniques to public health campaigns promoting exercise and nutrition, has added another layer of protection against what was once considered an inevitable fate for many Americans.

Yet despite these remarkable advances, one fundamental truth persists: lowering LDL cholesterol remains our most powerful weapon against heart disease. The science supporting this approach has only grown stronger over the decades, reinforced by countless studies and clinical observations that form an irrefutable body of evidence. As our understanding deepens, the central role of LDL cholesterol in cardiovascular disease becomes increasingly clear.

LDL cholesterol—often called the "silent architect" of arterial disease—orchestrates the gradual accumulation of plaque within our vessels, narrowing these vital pathways and setting the stage for heart attacks and strokes. This process, atherosclerosis, begins stealthily, often decades before symptoms appear. By the time chest pain or shortness of breath signals a problem, the disease has frequently progressed to a dangerous stage. The science is unequivocal: reduce your LDL cholesterol, and you diminish your risk of these life-altering events.

In the decade since I first published *Cholesterol Down*, I've been deeply moved by the thousands of readers who have shared their success stories. I hear from a great many people who have discovered they can take control of their cholesterol naturally, without necessarily resorting to medications. Their testimonials arrive in my inbox weekly—stories of individuals who followed the program and watched their LDL numbers drop by 30, 40, even 50 points. With the enhanced strategies in this revised edition, even more dramatic improvements are now possible.

What makes these successes particularly remarkable is that they were achieved through accessible, natural methods. The Cholesterol Down approach doesn't require expensive equipment, exotic ingredients, or complicated regimens. Instead, it harnesses the power of simple dietary additions, moderate lifestyle adjustments, and evidence-based natural compounds that work synergistically to improve blood cholesterol levels. This accessibility has democratized heart health, proving that significant cholesterol reduction isn't a privilege reserved for those with abundant resources or medical access—it's achievable for virtually anyone willing to implement these strategies consistently.

Though the core science behind the original Cholesterol Down program stands firm, our understanding of cardiovascular health continues to evolve at a breathtaking pace, enabling me to create an even more powerful LDL-lowering lifestyle strategy than was possible a decade ago. The last decade has brought remarkable insights into the role of inflammation in heart disease and the varying impacts of different dietary patterns on cholesterol metabolism. We now have a deeper understanding of how excess body fat affects cardiovascular function. Perhaps most importantly, we've accumulated stronger evidence about which natural approaches yield the most significant benefits for cholesterol management.

This revised edition incorporates these latest research findings and refined approaches that have emerged over the past decade. Most significantly, I've replaced an entire chapter with a more potent LDL-lowering strategy supported by compelling new scientific evidence: calorie restriction. You'll also find updated recommendations on optimal intake levels for plant sterols, the latest on soluble fiber's mechanisms of action, and new scientific data supporting the concept that combining certain foods can amplify their cholesterol-lowering effects. Recognizing that overweight and obesity are intimately tied to higher cholesterol levels, I provide simple, practical nutritional advice on eating healthy and weight loss. I've included a deep dive into the remarkable effect that losing body fat has on LDL cholesterol and offer a balanced perspective on the latest GLP-1 weight loss medications and their potential role in cardiovascular health.

The strategies I present aren't merely theoretical—they're proven pathways to better heart health that have already transformed countless lives. Unlike fad diets or trendy supplements that promise miraculous results without scientific backing, every recommendation in this book is grounded in peer-reviewed research and clinical experience. I've carefully evaluated the evidence, separating well-established findings from preliminary research, giving you clarity about what's definitively known versus what's still being investigated.

What distinguishes this approach from conventional medical management isn't opposition to medication but its emphasis on natural methods as either an alternative or a complement to drug therapy. Statins and other pharmaceuticals play a crucial role for many people, but for some readers, this program has allowed them to avoid medication entirely. For others, it has enabled them to reduce their dosage or enhance the effectiveness of their prescribed regimen. The goal isn't to replace medical care but to expand our arsenal of effective strategies for controlling cholesterol.

This new edition also addresses the evolving landscape of heart disease risk factors. While LDL cholesterol remains central to cardiovascular risk, we now recognize that other factors—triglyceride levels and inflammation markers—also play significant roles. I've incorporated targeted strategies for addressing these additional factors, creating a more comprehensive approach to heart health that extends beyond simple LDL reduction. The relationship between body composition and cholesterol levels receives special attention, reflecting groundbreaking research on how modest weight loss can dramatically improve your lipid panel.

As you embark on this journey through these pages, remember that knowledge alone doesn't change health outcomes—only action does. The information contained here isn't just about understanding cholesterol; it's about empowering you with practical, natural strategies to transform your cardiovascular health and potentially add vibrant years to your life. Each step you take—adding psyllium to your morning routine, incorporating more beans into your diet, or taking a daily walk—represents a small victory in your personal battle against heart disease.

The path to lower cholesterol isn't always easy, but it's undeniably worthwhile. The choices you make today will echo through the years ahead, potentially sparing you and your loved ones from the devastation that cardiovascular disease can bring. As someone who has dedicated my career to this field, I can assure you that few health investments yield greater returns than protecting your heart.

Welcome to the new edition of *Cholesterol Down*. Your heart's future may well depend on what you discover within these pages—pages that now contain an even more powerful approach to naturally lowering your LDL cholesterol and protecting your cardiovascular health.

INTRODUCTION

My father died prematurely of a heart attack, so when my doctor told me during a routine physical examination in 2004 that my LDL or "bad" cholesterol had reached a dangerously high level, I had cause for immediate concern.

As a nutritionist and marathon runner with an active lifestyle and healthy plant-based diet, I was shocked to find myself among the 105 million Americans who suffer from high cholesterol. Furthermore, as a woman, I assumed my gender would protect me—at least until after menopause. But the truth is that no one is safe. Genes as much as lifestyle factor into cholesterol levels, and everyone is vulnerable.

Statin drugs are the most common treatment for rapidly reducing cholesterol—though they are notorious for their safety concerns and long list of potential side effects, confirmed to me in many anecdotes told by my patients over the years. I've always been reluctant to take prescription medicines, and when my doctor suggested that I begin statin treatment immediately, I knew there had to be a better way—a healthier, drug-free plan for lowering LDL cholesterol.

So I began developing a diet and exercise prescription, based on a mixture of foods scientifically proven to effectively lower LDL cholesterol, experimenting on myself and willing patients. I was amazed to find that after several months on this program, my "bad" cholesterol had dropped from 160 mg/dL to 107 mg/dL, a 33 percent reduction! Further research revealed that even a remarkably short four-week time frame was sufficient to promote a significant drop in LDL cholesterol.

Several of my patients tried my four-week plan with incredible results. One patient lowered her LDL cholesterol 71 points, from 211 mg/dL to 140 mg/dL (a 34 percent reduction). A young man with a strong family history of heart disease lowered his "bad" cholesterol from 150 mg/dL to 80 mg/dL (an astonishing 47 percent drop in LDL cholesterol). These results are comparable to those achieved after a starting dose of a statin drug—only without the side effects.

This safe and easy-to-follow plan has yielded such miraculous results that I decided to write a how-to book that others could benefit from. *Cholesterol Down* is the result—a clear, practical, drug-free cholesterol-lowering plan based on solid scientific research.

STATIN DRUGS: WHAT ARE THE SIDE EFFECTS?

"My muscles and joints ached so much that I couldn't get out of bed and walk across the room! My doctor took me off Lipitor and tried two more statin drugs, but I just couldn't stand the side effects." A patient shared this story with me, driving home the fact that some individuals do experience intolerable side effects from taking statin drugs. Here is a list of the most commonly reported adverse side effects:

- Headache.
- Gastrointestinal complaints (nausea, upset stomach, diarrhea, constipation).
- Fatigue, flu-like symptoms.
- Elevated liver enzymes called transaminases (a potentially serious side effect).
- Myalgia. Muscle soreness, weakness, or pain without an associated elevation of creatine kinase (a muscle enzyme detected in the bloodstream).
- Myopathy (severe myositis or inflammation of the muscle). Muscle aches or weakness with an associated elevation of creatine kinase.

- Rhabdomyolysis (serious myopathy). Muscle aches or weakness with a marked elevation of creatine kinase and other muscle enzymes. In addition, in this rare but severe and life-threatening side effect, the muscle cells break down and release myoglobin (a muscle protein) into the bloodstream. This can result in kidney malfunction and ultimately kidney failure.

Sources: Connie B. Newman et al., "Statin Safety and Associated Adverse Events: A Scientific Statement from the American Heart Association," *Arteriosclerosis, Thrombosis, and Vascular Biology* 39, no. 2 (February 2019): e38–e81.

WHO SHOULD GO ON THIS PLAN

This plan was designed for otherwise healthy adults who want to lower their LDL or "bad" cholesterol using a safe and effective drug-free approach. Others may already be taking prescription statin drugs but may not have reached their physician-recommended LDL goal level. The Cholesterol Down Plan is also ideal for these individuals, who should use it to supplement statin drugs in order to keep their dosages low enough to reduce the risk of dangerous side effects associated with higher statin doses. As an adjunct to statin therapy, the Cholesterol Down Plan can be very effective for those high-risk individuals who need to attain the new government-advocated ultra-low LDL goal.

HOW TO USE THIS BOOK

There are two main parts to this book. Part I (Chapters 1 through 3) provides the scientific background for the Cholesterol Down Plan and gives you a foundation for Part II, the diet section. Part I teaches you everything you need to know about cholesterol, your diet, and heart disease, and why targeting LDL cholesterol is the focus of the Cholesterol Down Plan. If science is not your cup of tea, simply skip to Part II, the diet section, to start bringing your cholesterol down now.

Part II (Chapters 4 through 13) lays out the ten steps, one step per chapter, of the Cholesterol Down Plan. Before you begin the plan, I suggest you read all the steps and pay particular attention to the caveats at the end of each chapter. After getting the go-ahead from your physician, begin by assessing your starting point: have your blood analyzed and obtain your initial LDL value. Make several photocopies of the Ten-Step Daily Checklist (see Appendix 1), purchase all the components, and you're ready to begin. Checking off your daily steps will help you reach your aim of getting in all ten steps every day. Retest your blood every four weeks to track your progress. Regarding the fiber steps, remember to build up *slowly* to prevent any gastrointestinal distress. Start with half the prescribed amounts and add a little more fiber into your diet each day. Also, be sure to drink plenty of fluids.

The Appendixes provide tools for helping you stick to the Cholesterol Down Plan. In addition to the Ten-Step Daily Checklist, there is a six-month LDL Cholesterol Progress Chart (Appendix 2), two weeks of sample menus (Appendix 3), healthy recipes incorporating the required foods in the plan (Appendix 4), and tools to help you calculate your own risk for heart disease (Appendix 5).

HOW THIS BOOK DIFFERS FROM OTHER CHOLESTEROL BOOKS

This book is unique in that it not only provides a clear, step-by-step plan outlining exactly what to do—what foods to eat and in what amounts and how to exercise and how much—in order to significantly lower your cholesterol, but it also gives you the scientific basis behind each step so you understand *why* the plan works and how each step of the plan lowers LDL cholesterol in a different way for the maximum cumulative effect.

Cholesterol Down is the culmination of my experience as a licensed dietitian, exercise physiologist, certified wellness coach, and cholesterol patient myself. Based on my own needs and those of my patients, it's extremely user-friendly and designed to make it easy for you to stay on track.

I hope that this book will be a powerful, potentially lifesaving tool for you and the millions of Americans who want a safer, natural alternative or supplement to statin drugs for getting LDL cholesterol down.

PART I

Everything You Need to Know About Cholesterol, LDL, and Heart Disease

CHAPTER 1

Cholesterol 101

> The doctor of the future will give no medicine, but will interest his patients in the care of the human frame, in diet, and in the cause and prevention of disease.
>
> —THOMAS ALVA EDISON, AMERICAN SCIENTIST AND INVENTOR (1847–1931)

CARDIOVASCULAR DISEASE: WILL IT BE YOUR CAUSE OF DEATH?

Odds are that you will die from some form of cardiovascular disease—our nation's deadliest epidemic—be it a heart attack, stroke, high blood pressure, or other disease of the heart and blood vessels. In the United States, one person dies from cardiovascular disease approximately every thirty-three seconds. Combine that overwhelming death toll with the staggering $422.3 billion estimated direct and indirect cost of cardiovascular disease for 2023, and you begin to grasp the magnitude of this huge public health concern.[1]

More fearful that you will die of cancer? Recent American Heart Association statistics reveal that you are much more likely to succumb to a disease of the heart or blood vessels.[2] Currently, more than twice as many Americans die of cardiovascular disease than of cancer. In fact, cardiovascular disease claims more lives than the next four leading causes—cancer, respiratory diseases, accidents, and diabetes—combined.

If you are a woman and think your gender will protect you, you should know that in 2023 almost half a million American women died of cardiovascular disease, mainly heart disease. In fact, according to the American Heart Association's 2024 statistics, a woman's odds of dying from heart disease far surpassed her chances of dying from breast cancer (1 in 30 women who died did so of breast cancer, while 1 in 2.6 died of cardiovascular disease). Furthermore, more women succumbed to cardiovascular disease than men—approximately fifty thousand more women than men. The truth is that women are different from men, both in the symptoms of heart disease that women exhibit and in the propensity of women to exhibit a different but just as deadly type of heart disease, "coronary microvascular disease," which is a hardening of the minute arteries that feed the heart (they are too tiny to show up on a typical angiogram). According to new findings, high cholesterol and high blood pressure are among the leading causes of this condition.[3]

The good news is that lifestyle modifications will provide you with a powerful measure of protection against diseases of the heart and blood vessels, including microvascular disease. By following the easy ten-step Cholesterol Down Plan outlined in Part II of this book, you can lower your "bad" cholesterol—and maybe even save your life.

According to the World Health Organization's report *Global Strategy on Diet, Physical Activity, and Health,* various forms of cardiovascular disease resulted in an estimated 17.9 million deaths globally in 2019, representing 32 percent of all global deaths. Of these deaths, 85 percent were due to heart attack and stroke.

Source: "Cardiovascular Diseases (CVDs)," World Health Organization, July 31, 2025, www.who.int/news-room/fact-sheets/detail/cardiovascular-diseases-(cvds).

WHAT CAUSES A HEART ATTACK OR STROKE?

A heart attack or stroke is ultimately caused by a corroding of LDL particles that accumulate within the inner arterial wall, resulting in inflammation and eventual thickening of the arterial walls leading to the heart or brain, a process called atherosclerosis. This slow, progressive disease typically starts in childhood, when cholesterol, cellular debris, fat, calcium, and other compounds begin building up in the large arteries. Over time, a poor diet and sedentary lifestyle predispose our arteries to clogging up with this thick mass of gunk, called plaque, often with fatal consequences. Eventually the plaque ruptures and a blood clot forms; the flow of blood, oxygen, and nutrients is blocked, and a heart attack or stroke ensues.

Fortunately, there are a number of simple lifestyle changes that can protect your arteries from atherosclerosis. In later chapters, you will see how the Cholesterol Down Plan works to dramatically cut your cholesterol and reduce your chances of developing cardiovascular disease, including atherosclerosis.

Where Your Body Stores Cholesterol

Cells. Over 90 percent of all the cholesterol in the body is found in cell membranes. A great deal of cholesterol is also located in the nervous system, concentrated in the cells of the brain and spinal cord.

Liver. Huge amounts of cholesterol are found in the liver as a main component of bile, the digestive juice produced by the liver and stored in the gallbladder.

Steroid hormones. Cholesterol is a primary structural element of steroid hormones such as cortisol and aldosterone and the sex hormones, so a high concentration of cholesterol is found in the glands where these products are synthesized. Cholesterol allows women to be feminine and men to be masculine—it's a building block of the sex hormones estrogen and testosterone.

Bloodstream. Cholesterol is found in the bloodstream as "blood cholesterol" in small circular packages called lipoproteins.

WHAT IS CHOLESTEROL, ANYWAY?

Everyone talks about cholesterol, but few people actually understand what it is. In physical terms, it is a white fat-like substance with a consistency like candle wax that can be found nearly everywhere in the body: in the membranes of all cells, in the bile stored in the liver, in steroid hormones, and—most important for the purposes of this book—floating through the bloodstream in transport vehicles known as lipoproteins. Despite its bad rap, some cholesterol is vitally important for good health, as it is a major building block for many structures within our bodies—even our bones and teeth, as cholesterol is a precursor for vitamin D.

THE CHOLESTEROL TRANSIT SYSTEM

Oil doesn't mix with water, so it shouldn't be a surprise that oily cholesterol doesn't mix with blood, which is basically salty water. The body solves this problem by producing waterproof cholesterol transporters called lipoproteins. In addition to cholesterol, lipoproteins also ferry around dietary fat (known in scientific circles as triglyceride or triacylglycerol) and the fat-soluble vitamins E, D, A, and K. If you were to assemble a lipoprotein, you would need four building blocks: protein, cholesterol, triglycerides, and phospholipids (another type of waxy fat-like material found in high concentration in cell membranes). The amount of each substance varies depending on the class of lipoprotein.

THE FOUR TYPES OF LIPOPROTEINS

Lipoproteins are divided into four main classes according to density: chylomicrons, VLDL, LDL, and HDL (Figure 1.1). Lower-density lipoproteins are characterized by a higher fat-to-protein ratio (fat is lighter) and therefore float more easily in the blood. Here are the basics about the four classes of lipoproteins, in order of increasing density.

- **Chylomicrons** are the least dense of all the lipoproteins and are basically just big balls of fat (triglycerides), with a makeup of about 90 percent fat, a touch of phospholipids, some cholesterol, and a smidgen of protein.
- **VLDL** (very low-density lipoprotein) carries a great amount of fat, some phospholipids, and cholesterol. The high fat content of VLDL makes a large quantity of this lipoprotein in the blood undesirable.
- **LDL** (low-density lipoprotein, or "bad" cholesterol) has only a fraction of the fat and double the percentage of protein of VLDL and is very high in cholesterol. This lipoprotein carries the majority of cholesterol in the blood and is considered the unhealthy one.
- **HDL** (high-density lipoprotein, or "good" cholesterol) is a spherical blob of mostly protein (albeit a type different from that found in LDL), some cholesterol, phospholipids, and very little fat. The densest of all the lipoproteins, HDL is the healthy one.

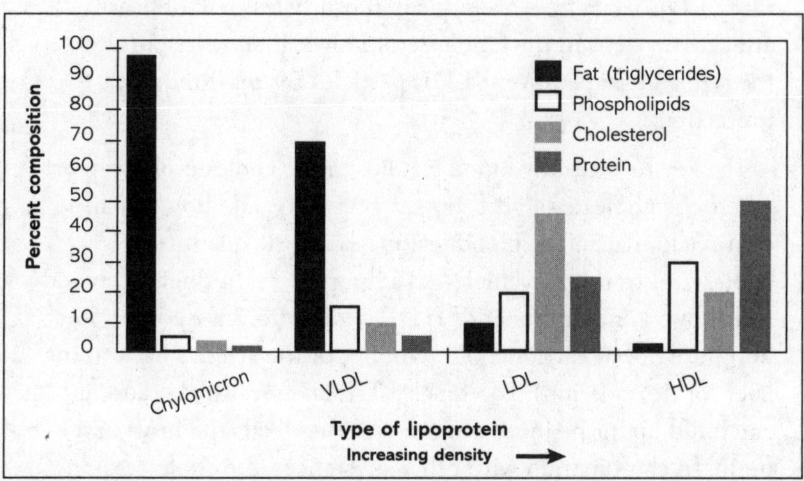

Figure 1.1. The four lipoproteins—chylomicrons, VLDL, LDL, and HDL—differ in composition.

MEASURING YOUR CHOLESTEROL

Your doctor will ask you to fast overnight before having your blood drawn to measure your lipoprotein levels. Fasting ensures that the chylomicrons are gone and have no effect on the sum total of cholesterol or triglycerides swimming around your bloodstream. The lab report will analyze your blood specimen for HDL, LDL, and VLDL. It will show the amount of "good" cholesterol (HDL), "bad" cholesterol (LDL), and triglycerides (blood fat) in the bloodstream. Your doctor may also test you for some risky particle characteristics—such as small and dense LDLs, small HDLs, or big VLDL particles—if you are at high risk for heart disease.

When It Comes to LDL, Size Matters

The most dangerous situation is when cholesterol is transported in a barrage of small, dense LDL particles that can slip through the cracks and congregate within the arterial wall. Numerous studies have shown that when one reverses the lipoprotein transport patterns—from a dangerous pattern of small, heavy LDL particles to a heart-healthy pattern of very few large and fluffy LDL particles—there is significantly less risk of heart attack. The steps in the Cholesterol Down Plan will help alter the size and shape of your LDL particles for maximum heart protection.

The key to a healthy blood test lies in the cholesterol transport: where the cholesterol goes, how it gets there, and how much of it accumulates. The blood test measures the quantity of cholesterol transport vehicles (aka lipoproteins). A healthy blood test shows a high number of HDL cholesterol transporters (the lipoprotein that carries cholesterol out of the arteries back to the liver for degradation). Too much LDL is unhealthy because it can build up in the inner arterial wall that feeds the heart and brain. In combination with other substances, the cholesterol in LDL forms plaque, which clogs the arteries (atherosclerosis).

If a blood clot forms, cells downstream die, and a heart attack or stroke occurs. Atherosclerosis is therefore a disease process related to problems with cholesterol transport.

Numbers Your Doctor Will Be Concerned About

- **High total cholesterol.** This number reflects the total amount of cholesterol found in all the lipoproteins (LDL, HDL, VLDL) circulating in the blood. According to the American Heart Association, *a value of less than 200 mg/dL is desirable for a relatively low risk of heart disease.*

- **Low HDL.** To keep your heart and blood vessels in top shape, it is beneficial to have as high a concentration of HDL particles in the blood as possible. Too low an amount is unhealthy. According to the American Heart Association, *a value of less than 40 mg/dL heightens your risk of heart disease.*

- **High LDL.** The higher your LDL, the higher your risk of heart and vessel disease. As you shall learn, LDL is the most telltale sign of risk. According to the American Heart Association, *an optimal level of LDL cholesterol is less than 100 mg/dL.* (See Chapter 2 for an in-depth discussion of why high LDL is so risky.)

- **High triglyceride.** Your triglyceride value reflects the amount of blood fats circulating. A high number is also a risk factor for heart disease. According to the American Heart Association, *a normal triglyceride level is less than 150 mg/dL.*

- **High ratio of total cholesterol to HDL.** Some physicians use the ratio of total cholesterol to HDL cholesterol to determine risk for heart disease. A high number means there is too little "good" cholesterol and too much "bad" cholesterol. According to the American Heart Association, *the optimal ratio is 3.5:1 or less.*

Source: "What Your Cholesterol Levels Mean," American Heart Association, February 16, 2024, www.heart.org/en/health-topics/cholesterol/about-cholesterol/what-your-cholesterol-levels-mean.

HDL, THE LIFESAVING LIPOPROTEIN

HDL is manufactured in the small intestine and the liver, its primary source. As it moves through the bloodstream, it takes in excess cholesterol that leaches out of tissue cells and, most important, excess cholesterol building up in the inner arterial wall. HDLs unload this cholesterol in the liver, where it is then excreted via bile, a process referred to as "reverse cholesterol transport." Other lipoproteins bring cholesterol into the cells, so it is this reverse transport from the cells to the liver that distinguishes HDL as the "good" cholesterol. An elevated level of HDL has been associated with a reduced risk for heart disease. HDL confers heart-protective benefits in four ways.

1. HDL circulates around the body, picking up excess cholesterol and bringing it back to the liver for disposal (reverse cholesterol transport).

2. HDL is an antioxidant, capable of dismantling rogue free radical molecules that oxidize the protein in the LDL particles—a contributing factor to atherosclerosis. (Oxidation is the same process that produces rust on metals.)

3. HDL exhibits anti-inflammatory activity (like aspirin) and can decrease the inflammation linked with the atherosclerotic process.

4. HDL lessens the ability of the blood to form clots, thus reducing the risk of heart attack or stroke.

 HDL vs. LDL: A Comparison

	HDL ("Good" Cholesterol)	LDL ("Bad" Cholesterol)
What it is composed of	Mostly protein, some cholesterol and phospholipids, very little fat	Mostly cholesterol, a moderate quantity of protein and phospholipids, and some fat
Where it is produced	Almost all HDL is formed in liver cells, with a small quantity produced by intestinal cells	Cells of the liver and intestine produce VLDL; LDL evolves from VLDL
Where it is found	In the bloodstream and inner arterial wall	In the bloodstream and inner arterial wall
Direction of transport	From the cells of the body to the liver	Initially from the liver (as VLDL) to all cells throughout the body
Effect on the arteries leading to the heart and brain	Protects against the development of atherosclerosis	Promotes the development of atherosclerosis
Effect of quantity on heart health	Low amount is a risk factor for heart disease	High amount is a risk factor for heart disease
Optimal particle size	Larger-sized HDL particles (HDL2b) are most protective (indicating active reverse cholesterol transport)	Larger-sized LDL particles are desirable, as small, dense LDL particles increase risk of atherosclerosis
Optimal amount	Greater than 40 mg/dL; the higher the better	Less than 100 mg/dL; the lower the better

LDL, THE DEADLY LIPOPROTEIN

LDL is the chief cholesterol carrier in the blood, ferrying approximately 70 percent of the body's blood cholesterol around the network of arteries. Basically, this lipoprotein is loaded with cholesterol. Unlike HDL, LDL is not directly manufactured in the liver. Instead, a different type of lipoprotein is first produced by the liver, the parent lipoprotein called VLDL. After circulating around the bloodstream, VLDL loses much of its fat (triglyceride) cache to various bodily cells to become LDL. LDL is designed to take cholesterol to cells that have run short, as cells require some cholesterol to maintain proper functioning. Typically, the LDL is taken into the cell and broken down, and then the cholesterol is used to make membranes or hormones. However, when the amount of LDL in the blood gets too high, the situation can become injurious.

WHY IS LDL SO DANGEROUS?

LDL is commonly referred to as the "bad" cholesterol because high levels of circulating LDL have been linked to an increased risk for atherosclerosis and cardiovascular disease. LDL is the most dangerous lipoprotein, not only because each particle is made up of mostly cholesterol (roughly 45 percent) but also because of its destination. LDL carries cholesterol to the arteries, infiltrates their walls, and goes through a series of transformations that trigger plaque buildup.

WHAT DOES THIS "BAD" CHOLESTEROL LOOK LIKE?

LDL cholesterol is a round lipoprotein that shuttles the bulk of the cholesterol in the blood. The inner core contains oily cholesterol molecules, each with a fatty acid chain dangling from it. Also found within the core is a lesser amount of triglyceride molecules intermingling with the cholesterol esters. Seventy-five percent of the cholesterol within the LDL is in this bound-up (esterified) form, concentrated within the inner core. The greater the concentration of these "chained" cholesterol molecules in the LDL, the more susceptible the LDL molecule is to oxidation (which instigates the catastrophic events that make up the atherosclerotic process) and the higher your risk for developing heart disease.

Low-density lipoprotein

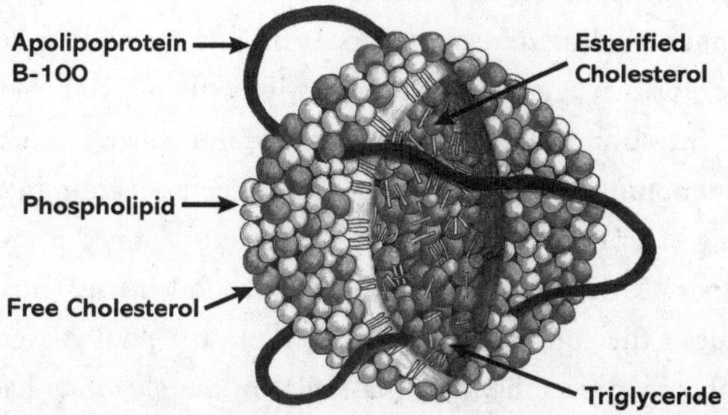

Figure 1.2. LDL cholesterol is a round lipoprotein that exists in several different sizes. LDL shuttles the bulk of the cholesterol in the blood.

Surrounding the fatty core of LDL is an outer shell consisting of many fat-like molecules called phospholipids plus some "unchained" cholesterol. The entire LDL ball is encircled by one big spaghetti-like strand of protein called Apo B (apolipoprotein B-100) (Figure 1.2). This protein molecule plays a crucial role in mooring the LDL molecule onto LDL receptors (more on these later).

EATING YOUR WAY TO A HEART ATTACK

What most people don't realize is that cholesterol comes from two sources: from food and from our own cells. In fact, we actually make three times more cholesterol (about 1,000–1,200 mg per day) than we typically eat. So we don't need to eat cholesterol because the body is perfectly capable of manufacturing enough of this waxy substance on its own. Still, Americans continue to consume an appreciable amount of cholesterol from dietary sources, which can raise "bad" cholesterol levels and increase our risk of heart disease. The average American ingests approximately 300–400 mg of cholesterol every day from animal sources. This amount exceeds the government's cholesterol-lowering dietary recommendation of no more than 200 mg a day. It is simple to eat this much cholesterol: seven ounces of liver (providing 762 mg of cholesterol) or two egg yolks (424 mg) will easily put you over the top.

In the intestine is a reservoir of cholesterol called the cholesterol pool. The amount of cholesterol that enters the pool from bile is up to five times greater than the amount of cholesterol derived from our diet. Where does all that cholesterol floating around in the intestine go? About half of the approximately 2,000 mg in the pool is excreted and half is reabsorbed into the intestinal cells, ultimately going back to the liver. If you could block reabsorption of some of the cholesterol in the intestinal pool so that it gets excreted and not returned to the liver, then you would decrease your circulating LDL level. One class of cholesterol-lowering drugs in particular capitalizes on this concept.

HOW IS CHOLESTEROL ABSORBED FROM THE INTESTINAL POOL INTO THE BODY?

For cholesterol, the gateway into the body is a layer of cells lining the upper intestine known as enterocytes. The only way for cholesterol to get to this layer is to attach itself to a transporter called a micelle. Micelles are small, round transport packages formed by bile salts and phospholipids that carry cholesterol and fat (triglycerides) to the intestinal cell wall. The cholesterol must then take a second transport route—a protein channel called Niemann-Pick C1 Like 1, or NPC1L1 for short.[4] The cholesterol enters the NPC1L1 channel, traverses through the wall and into the intestinal cell, where it is packaged into chylomicrons for travel in the lymph system and ultimately the bloodstream. Zetia, the cholesterol-lowering drug, blocks cholesterol absorption from the intestine by targeting the NPC1L1 protein.

Once in the bloodstream, chylomicrons off-load lots of triglycerides to needy cells, eventually arriving at the liver as small, cholesterol-rich particles known as chylomicron remnants. These remnants signal to the liver cells that they don't have to make more cholesterol, as a new cholesterol shipment has arrived—cholesterol that may have come from your breakfast omelet. The liver extracts the cholesterol from the remnants to make whatever is required for the day. Typically, the cholesterol is converted into bile acids for its launch into the body's cholesterol recycling system. But the liver could instead package the cholesterol up as a lipoprotein (primarily VLDL) and send it back into the bloodstream, ultimately increasing the amount of "bad" LDL cholesterol. Eat a huge amount of cholesterol and you increase the delivery of cholesterol to the liver by chylomicron remnants. Therefore, you should avoid foods with high cholesterol in order to lower the amount of cholesterol in your intestinal pool. Less cholesterol overloading the liver means less VLDL exported and less LDL produced.

THE LIVER, A CHOLESTEROL FACTORY

The liver is a glutton when it comes to cholesterol. Its cells work around the clock using huge amounts of cholesterol, mainly to manufacture ingredients in bile. In fact, almost 80 percent of the cholesterol in the liver is used to produce key ingredients in bile, which is secreted into the small intestine for fat digestion. The liver also uses cholesterol for lipoprotein production, particularly VLDL (the parent molecule of LDL). The foremost source of "bad" LDL cholesterol is the liver, which indirectly functions as an LDL production facility.

THE BODY'S CHOLESTEROL RECYCLING SYSTEM

Think of the liver as not only a bile and lipoprotein manufacturing plant but also a cholesterol removal and recycling plant. How does the liver recycle cholesterol? The liver cells build bile acids from cholesterol. The bile acids are then secreted in bile (along with free cholesterol) into the upper section of the small intestine, where they aid in fat digestion. Once in the acidic environment of the small intestine, the bile acids convert into bile salts. Bile salts are continuously recycled from the intestine and returned to the liver. Each bile salt is reused about twenty times before it is excreted out of the body in the feces.

The liver, therefore, doesn't need to churn out too much new "homemade" cholesterol because it has this neat recycling program (called enterohepatic circulation) in which the bile acids (formerly cholesterol) are continuously recycled between the intestines and the liver. Almost 95 percent of the bile acids entering the intestine are recirculated and absorbed back into the bloodstream, heading straight to the liver, where they are once again secreted into the intestine as bile. This recycling system decreases the liver's requirement for new cholesterol and inhibits its production of new bile acids from cholesterol.

How much cholesterol the liver uses up each day to make bile acids depends on the return flow of bile salts from the intestine. Sequestering bile salts in the intestine so that they are excreted in waste and not recycled will force the liver to increase LDL clearance from the blood to replenish the cells' internal cholesterol stores (used for making new key bile ingredients). Another class of cholesterol-lowering drugs works in this fashion. An important concept to keep in mind is that there is only one primary route out of the body for cholesterol (in the form of either free cholesterol or bile salts), and that is through the feces by way of the intestinal tract. If you block the absorption of free cholesterol or interrupt the recirculation of bile salts by trapping them in the intestine and excreting them, the end result is a drop in circulating LDL cholesterol. Several steps in the Cholesterol Down Plan work to lower LDL in this manner.

THE BODY'S MAIN LDL REGULATORY ORGAN

The liver is the only organ capable of breaking cholesterol down and getting rid of it via bile. It does this through receptors, the little vacuum-like protein tunnels that sprout out from the liver cell membranes and suck up the circulating LDL. Once inside, LDL is broken down, and the cholesterol is used mainly for building new bile acids, which are then excreted in bile out into the intestine. (Note that bile acid synthesis is the main route by which cholesterol is removed from the body.)

High LDL? Don't Blame It All on Genes

Some people do have the unfortunate luck of inheriting a genetic predisposition to make truckloads of cholesterol internally. Most LDL is removed from the circulation by LDL receptors on the liver. Certain individuals inherit a tendency to produce fewer receptors, resulting in less LDL removal from the blood (predisposing them to excess LDL and atherosclerosis). With regard to receptors, we can't blame it all on the genes. The food you eat can greatly affect the density of the receptors on the liver. Ingestion of dietary cholesterol, saturated fat, and trans fat has unhealthy consequences. These foods suppress the manufacturing of cholesterol-clearing liver receptors and raise your "bad" cholesterol level. For a one-two punch against heart disease, eat a heart-healthy diet (low in saturated fat and cholesterol and devoid of trans fat) and follow the Cholesterol Down Plan, which includes foods that help augment the number of LDL receptors.

By clearing excess LDL from the bloodstream, LDL receptors help protect against atherosclerosis.[5] After the liver, the cells of the adrenal gland and ovaries have the most receptors because these are the cells in the body with the greatest need for cholesterol. Any agent or medication capable of increasing the number of receptors on the liver cells will reduce the concentration of blood-borne "bad" LDL cholesterol. The density of LDL receptors plays a critical role in atherosclerosis. The fewer LDL receptors you have on your liver, the more circulating LDL particles and the greater your risk of heart disease.

You now understand the basics of cholesterol mechanics and the importance of maintaining normal lipoprotein levels in your bloodstream. The ten simple steps in the Cholesterol Down Plan capitalize on the ability of certain foods plus exercise to exploit the body's LDL-lowering mechanisms in order to promote heart health and prevent the development or recurrence of heart and blood vessel disease.

CHAPTER 2

Targeting LDL

"My doctor says my 'bad' cholesterol is too low—is this good or bad?"

"You mean your 'good' cholesterol is too low, right?"

"Yes, I guess so. Can you please explain to me which cholesterol numbers I need to know?"

My patients routinely hand me the blood work printout they received from their doctor and ask me to translate the numbers, as they are baffled by the alphabet soup associated with heart health. True, there are myriad factors that increase your risk for heart disease, such as family history, smoking, and high blood pressure. Other factors that increase your risk will be evident from your blood work: high total cholesterol, low HDL cholesterol, high LDL, high triglycerides, a high ratio of total cholesterol to HDL, a high number of small, dense LDL particles, and so on.

THE MOST IMPORTANT NUMBER: LDL

To streamline an otherwise complex topic for my patients, and for the purposes of this book, I recommend (with loads of science to substantiate this approach) that you familiarize yourself with one particular number above even your total cholesterol number—the "bad," LDL cholesterol—and leave the remaining values for your primary care physician to interpret. Learning to pay attention to this one number will not only make things easier, it will give you greater control in monitoring your risk for heart disease. If tracked over time, your LDL cholesterol will provide you with a clear and highly motivating snapshot of how your lifestyle changes are positively affecting you.

WHAT IS THE RATIONALE FOR TARGETING LDL?

There are five strong arguments for targeting LDL: (1) It is just plain easier to focus on one representative number. Like stepping on a scale to check your progress on a weight loss program, measuring LDL helps you assess your cholesterol level. (2) The nation's top two heart health agencies—the American Heart Association and the National Heart, Lung, and Blood Institute—specify lowering LDL as the primary therapeutic aim for individuals with high cholesterol. (3) Decades of scientific evidence derived from both human population studies and animal research demonstrate a link among high cholesterol, high LDL cholesterol, and heart disease. (4) Two Nobel Prize–winning scientists, Michael S. Brown and Joseph L. Goldstein, demonstrated the danger caused by too much circulating LDL in the blood. (5) Recent intervention studies utilizing powerful statin drugs have shown that lowering LDL saves lives, prevents new heart problems, and even reverses plaque buildup.

KEEP IT SIMPLE

The most obvious reason to focus on LDL cholesterol is that it is simpler to track one representative value rather than wade through all the values associated with heart disease.

Equate this concept with losing weight and stepping on a scale. One could analyze the percentage of body fat, calculate body mass index, or take circumferential measurements to reflect change in body composition. Most of my patients don't want to do that. They prefer the easiest and quickest method of getting feedback regarding the efficacy of their weight loss efforts: stepping on a scale. One, two, three . . . they either lost weight or they didn't! I tell them to weigh themselves once a week and let me do the rest of the calculations.

The same can be said for cholesterol: focus on your LDL cholesterol number and let your physician test for and interpret the myriad of additional values associated with your risk for cardiovascular disease. Targeting and reducing your LDL cholesterol number will diminish your chances of cardiovascular disease, may even shrink plaque buildup, and will help stabilize vulnerable plaque if the process of atherosclerosis has already advanced to this precarious stage in your arteries.

Above all else, you must know your LDL number and understand that with lifestyle changes, such as the Cholesterol Down Plan, this is a number you can control and lower to reduce your risk for cardiovascular disease. Appendix 2 is an LDL Cholesterol Progress Chart that makes it simple to track your LDL value as it decreases over each four-week interval, along with your odds of heart disease, when you follow the Cholesterol Down Plan.

HEART HEALTH AGENCIES COME DOWN ON LDL

In 1985, amid an epidemic of cardiovascular disease in the United States, the government's National Heart, Lung, and Blood Institute (a division of the National Institutes of Health) mounted an aggressive campaign to educate the public about the connection between high blood cholesterol and heart disease, called the National Cholesterol Education Program (NCEP). NCEP has clearly succeeded in its goal of educating Americans about the health risk of high blood cholesterol. What's needed now is a clear and concise message that *the LDL cholesterol value is the single most important number for the public to know.*

To increase citizens' awareness of the danger associated with high LDL, several of the nation's top heart health agencies have stated in their official guidelines that reducing LDL cholesterol is associated with reduced risk for heart disease.

A paragraph in the NCEP patient handout "Cholesterol & Your Heart: What You Need to Know" reads: "The main goal in treating high cholesterol is to lower your LDL or 'bad' cholesterol level."[1]

WHAT THE TOP DOGS HAVE TO SAY

In 1988, NCEP convened an expert panel that set out to review the latest scientific data and publish a report containing treatment recommendations for physicians. This report, titled *Detection, Evaluation, and Treatment of High Blood Cholesterol in Adults* (or ATP I), became the bible for determining how doctors should categorize and treat their patients at risk for heart disease and stroke. According to the most recent cholesterol guidelines, "LDL has long been identified as the primary target of cholesterol-lowering therapy," a focus that "has been strongly validated by recent clinical trials" in that they have shown that significantly lowering LDL indeed reduces the risk for coronary heart disease. In addition, "a broad base of evidence indicates that elevations in LDL cholesterol are a direct cause of atherosclerosis. Long-term elevations of LDL lead to a progressive accumulation of coronary atherosclerosis," which is a precursor to heart attacks or stroke.[2]

According to the newer ATP III panel guidelines, "all ATP reports have identified low-density lipoprotein cholesterol (LDL-C) as the primary target of cholesterol-lowering therapy," a statement supported by many large-scale studies that clearly show that a high amount of LDL in the blood is "a major risk factor for coronary heart disease (CHD)."[3] Furthermore, a large number of smaller intervention studies have documented that lowering the amount of LDL in the bloodstream reduces the risk of a major heart attack.

The American Heart Association 2021 Scientific Statement, Dietary Guidance to Improve Cardiovascular Health, concurs with NCEP, warning that "high total and LDL cholesterol levels are strongly related to coronary artery disease risk and . . . reductions in LDL levels are associated with reduced coronary disease risk." The American Heart Association further recommends that all Americans take "dietary measures aimed at maintaining desirable LDL cholesterol levels, as defined by the current guidelines of the National Cholesterol Education Program (NCEP)."[4]

ATP IV VERSUS ATP III½

The government published an update to the 2001 ATP III report, familiarly known in scientific circles as "ATP III½." The update included a "very high risk" category as well as a record ultra-low LDL target for those individuals in this category (LDL less than 70 mg/dL).[5] Since then, the American College of Cardiology (ACC) and the American Heart Association (AHA) has released new guidelines for treatment of high blood cholesterol, often referred to as ATP IV. These guidelines were designed to update the previous Adult Treatment Panel III (ATP III) report of the National Cholesterol Education Program (NCEP).

Although there are similarities between ATP III and the ACC/AHA guidelines, the two are fundamentally different. ATP III summarizes several decades of research on the relationship between LDL cholesterol and the process of atherosclerosis. It is based on the concept that lowering atherogenic lipoproteins (LDL cholesterol) will prevent heart disease. ACC/AHA guidelines, on the other hand, have been transformed into statin treatment instructions. They give lip service to lifestyle intervention without stating the clear scientific evidence supporting lifestyle intervention as the primary strategy for preventing and treating heart disease. The Cholesterol Down Plan stands by the original ATP III recommendations.

The Cholesterol Down Plan can be very useful for people in this highest-risk category as an adjunct to statin treatment. I've included the most therapeutic dose for some of the steps that will aid you in reaching this ultra-low LDL target.

SCIENCE LINKS HIGH LDL CHOLESTEROL WITH HEART DISEASE

Another argument that supports targeting LDL as the focal point for preventing cardiovascular disease lies with Michael S. Brown and Joseph L. Goldstein's revolutionary contribution to the understanding of how cholesterol is regulated in the body.

Brown and Goldstein discovered small proteins located on cell surfaces that function to take up circulating LDL from the bloodstream. They revealed details of the intricate connection among LDL receptors, the level of circulating LDL cholesterol, and the risk of atherosclerosis. If you recall, LDL receptors (located primarily on the surface of liver cells) help clear LDL from the bloodstream. Therefore, the greater the number of receptors, the lower the blood level of LDL. In 1984, Brown and Goldstein reported their groundbreaking discovery in *Scientific American:* "The LDL receptor hypothesis states that much of the atherosclerosis in the general population is caused by a dangerously high blood level of LDL resulting from failure to produce enough LDL receptors."[6] The next year, they received the Nobel Prize in Physiology or Medicine for elucidating the role of LDL receptors in cholesterol metabolism and the atherosclerotic process.

Building on their work, researchers have since been able to identify ways to increase the production of LDL receptors. In fact, several of the foods in the Cholesterol Down Plan help fight LDL by affecting these receptors. Eating almonds, for instance, helps increase the affinity of LDL particles for the receptors, and in test-tube experiments, an extract of Red Delicious apples has been shown to stimulate the growth of more LDL receptors on liver cells. Similarly, soy protein and its associated isoflavones were found to increase the production of LDL receptors in cells, which significantly lowers LDL cholesterol.[7] The bottom line: increasing LDL receptors lowers your "bad" LDL cholesterol and is as easy as following the Cholesterol Down Plan.

Over the past several decades, scientific studies have continued to yield results supporting the fact that high LDL is the principal contributing factor in the development of atherosclerosis. Relevant research ranges from large-scale population studies (epidemiological research) to clinical intervention (such as studies showing that lowering LDL by means of powerful statin medications reduces heart disease) and animal research.

LARGE-SCALE RESEARCH

Data derived from large-scale studies across different populations (comparing people from different countries, known as epidemiological research) shows that the higher the cholesterol level, the greater the degree of atherosclerosis evident in the population. This type of research illustrates that countries such as the United States—where the average LDL level has been estimated at approximately 123 mg/dL—have higher rates of heart disease than countries with lower average LDL numbers *(under 100 mg/dL is considered by the American Heart Association as an optimal goal for most individuals)*.

In 1994, two British scientists, Malcolm Law and Nicholas Wald, compiled an in-depth data analysis of the relationship between blood cholesterol level and rates of heart disease. Law and Wald estimated the average total cholesterol level of individuals residing in seventeen different countries over a forty-year time period and found tremendous variability: from 147 mg/dL (rural China) to 270 mg/dL (Finland) *(a total cholesterol value of under 200 mg/dL is considered optimal by the American Heart Association)*.[8] The three main conclusions were: the countries with the highest cholesterol levels had the greatest risk for heart disease; the increase in risk is specifically associated with an elevation in LDL cholesterol, which is determined by diet; and a difference in total cholesterol or LDL of just 23 mg/dL between countries is associated with a mean difference in death rates of 37 percent.

Another classic large-scale study, the famed "Seven Countries Study," provides additional support for the contention that high LDL cholesterol is firmly linked to the development of heart disease.[9] Pioneering nutrition researcher Ancel Keys analyzed and compared the diet and lifestyles of thousands of people living in Finland, Italy, Greece, the Netherlands, Japan, the United States, and Yugoslavia from 1958 to 1970. The data revealed that in countries where people consumed a diet high in saturated fat, there was a correspondingly high level of blood cholesterol and a significantly higher rate of heart attack and stroke. In fact, the death rate for heart disease in southern Europe (where the diet is low in saturated fat and the inhabitants have correspondingly low cholesterol levels) was half that of northern Europe and the United States. Thus, Keys's research revealed for the first time that risk of death from cardiovascular disease is strongly related to the level of saturated fat in the diet and the corresponding amount of blood cholesterol.

DATABASES OF AMERICAN COMMUNITIES

Ongoing studies of American communities have created enormously powerful databases that help scientists compile risk factors for the development of cardiovascular disease. Well-known studies such as the Multiple Risk Factor Intervention Trial (MRFIT), the Chicago Heart Association Detection Project in Industry (CHA), and the Peoples Gas Company Study (PG) have tracked thousands of Americans for years to find that a rise in cardiovascular disease risk is directly linked to high levels of blood cholesterol.

In an effort to ascertain the long-term impact of high cholesterol on risk of death from heart disease or other causes of death, scientists performed an analysis combining data from groups of younger men (eighteen to thirty-nine years at baseline) drawn from the MRFIT, CHA, and PG studies.[10] The men (approximately 80,000) were evaluated at baseline, and then cause of death was determined at the long-term follow-up, which differed among studies (twenty-five years for CHA, thirty-four years for PG, and sixteen years for MRFIT). The main findings were as follows: there was a strong relationship between high blood cholesterol level in younger men and long-term risk of death from heart disease, and young men with favorable total cholesterol values (<200 mg/dL) lived a substantially longer period of time (3.8 to 8.7 years longer) compared to those men with an initial total cholesterol level greater than 240 mg/dL. Note that although LDL was not recorded in these studies, a high total cholesterol value implies high LDL, as LDL carries the bulk of the cholesterol in the bloodstream.

Another large-scale study specifically examined the relationship between LDL cholesterol level and risk of heart disease.[11] Researchers from the National Heart, Lung, and Blood Institute recruited a total of 12,339 healthy, middle-aged men and women (forty-five to sixty-four years old) from communities in North Carolina, Mississippi, Minnesota, and Maryland to participate in the Atherosclerosis Risk in Communities Study (ARIC). Heart attacks and death from heart disease–related events were determined over a ten-year follow-up period. There was a strong association between high LDL cholesterol and risk of death. What's more, in both men and women, a much lower risk of death was observed in subjects with an LDL value of less than 100 mg/dL, prompting the researchers to categorize an LDL cholesterol value of less than 100 mg/dL as optimal.

Exciting data from the same ARIC study surfaced that graphically illustrate the dramatic lifelong benefit of even a moderate reduction in LDL levels.[12] A small percentage of the black volunteers had a genetic mutation that kept the LDL level of these particular subjects approximately 28 percent lower (average LDL was 100 mg/dL) than other study subjects (average LDL was 138 mg/dL). During the fifteen years of follow-up, only one of the 85 volunteers with the genetic mutation developed heart disease, compared to 10 percent of black subjects without the gene mutation. Remarkably, this 28 percent reduction in LDL translated into a reduction of almost 90 percent in the risk of heart disease. These results show the value of lowering your LDL level and keeping it down for life.

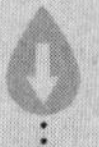

Reduce Your Risk

According to new research estimates, for every 1 percent reduction in LDL cholesterol, you reduce your risk of developing heart disease by approximately 2 percent. That means that *if you can get your LDL down from, say, 160 mg/dL to 120 mg/dL, you would cut your risk of a heart attack by more than half.*

Sources: Michael G. Silverman, "Association Between Lowering LDL-C and Cardiovascular Risk Reduction Among Different Therapeutic Interventions, A Systematic Review and Meta-Analysis," *JAMA* 316, no. 12 (2016): 1289–1297.

ANIMAL STUDIES

The data drawn from animal research also provide sufficient evidence to incriminate LDL as the main villain in heart disease. For instance, experimental animals fed a high-fat diet to induce an elevated level of circulating LDL exhibit high rates of atherosclerosis, similar to that of their human counterparts with high LDL levels.

In a classic study of diet-induced atherosclerosis in hamsters conducted by a group of Romanian researchers, male hamsters were fed a diet high in saturated fat and cholesterol.[13] After four weeks, their LDL shot up fourfold; after ten months, it had reached thirteen times the control hamsters' level. The resulting atherosclerotic process was immediately evident in the hamsters' aortas, where huge masses of plaque had amassed that would eventually lead to blood clots and, finally, heart attacks.

Another study in baboons showed that a diet high in cholesterol and saturated fat resulted in a significant elevation of LDL cholesterol.[14] Ten baboons were placed on the artery-clogging diet for a period of seven weeks. A section of the baboons' arteries was then surgically removed and examined microscopically. Along with the significant elevation of LDL cholesterol, researchers discovered severe inflammation within the arteries and evidence that a series of events termed "endothelial dysfunction" had occurred, a situation that promotes early atherosclerotic changes. Granted, hamsters are hamsters, baboons are baboons, and humans are humans, but the research shows that our bodies work similarly: across the board, increased levels of LDL mean an increased risk of atherosclerosis. For further evidence of the connection between the two, let's turn to compelling new findings taken from results of five large-scale scientific research studies employing statin drug therapy.[15]

STATIN STUDIES SHOW THE BENEFITS OF LOWER LDL

Each of these studies clearly demonstrates the health benefits of lowering LDL cholesterol to values well under the previous goal for high-risk patients of less than 100 mg/dL. In fact, they are what prompted the government to issue its ATP III½ revision, including the ultra-low LDL target. The five studies are the Heart Protection Study (HPS), the Prospective Study of Pravastatin in the Elderly at Risk (PROSPER), the Antihypertensive and Lipid-Lowering Treatment to Prevent Heart Attack Trial-Lipid Lowering Trial (ALLHAT-LLT), the Anglo-Scandinavian Cardiac Outcomes Trial-Lipid Lowering Arm (ASCOT-LLA), and the Pravastatin or Atorvastatin Evaluation and Infection-Thrombolysis in Myocardial Infarction (PROVE IT–TIMI 22).

THE FIVE STATIN MEGA-STUDIES: A CLOSER LOOK

HPS. This study took place in the United Kingdom and was carried out on 20,536 adults ages forty to eighty at high risk for a heart attack (subjects had a previous diagnosis of coronary artery disease or diabetes). Patients were prescribed either 40 mg per day of a statin drug called Zocor or given a placebo pill over a period of five years, after which researchers determined that Zocor reduced a patient's risk of heart attack and stroke by approximately 25 percent. The LDL cholesterol was lowered in the Zocor group from an initial average of less than 116 mg/dL to less than 77 mg/dL in one subsection of the statin group and from about 156 g/dL to 117 mg/dL in the other subsection. This study proved that lowering LDL cholesterol 25 to 34 percent with a statin drug is a highly effective means of preventing heart attacks and stroke in a high-risk population.

ALLHAT-LLT. This trial drew patients from 513 community clinics in North America (United States, Puerto Rico, Canada, and the U.S. Virgin Islands). A total of 10,355 people at high risk for heart disease, age fifty-five or older with moderately high LDL cholesterol and high blood pressure, were recruited and randomized to either treatment with the statin drug Pravachol (40 mg/day) or to a "usual care" group. For purposes of the study, "usual care" was defined as treatment for high LDL according to the discretion of the subject's primary physician, which could include statin therapy. After four years, researchers found that LDL declined from 146 mg/dL to 102 mg/dL in the Pravachol group compared to 146 mg/dL to 122 mg/dL in the "usual care" group. No significant difference between the two groups was observed in terms of measured outcome (death rate from coronary artery disease or heart attacks). The problem with this study was that only 70 percent of the Pravachol group complied with their medication treatment, and almost 30 percent in the "usual care" group took cholesterol-lowering drugs, factors that greatly diminished the ability to detect a difference between the two. However, the Pravachol group did exhibit an almost 10 percent reduction in heart attack risk; however, this finding did not reach statistical significance. This finding suggests that the 20-point-lower LDL number confers greater protection. The authors of the study concluded that despite the small difference in outcome between the two groups, the results are still consistent with findings from other large-scale statin studies: lowering LDL is vital for the prevention and treatment of heart disease. The lower the LDL, the greater the reduction in risk.

ASCOT-LLA. This large-scale European trial recruited patients from several Nordic countries as well as the United Kingdom and Ireland. Researchers tested the impact of Lipitor in 10,305 people with high blood pressure. Patients were divided into two groups, one that took 10 mg of Lipitor per day and another that took a placebo. After just one year, and compared to the placebo group, the Lipitor group had an LDL cholesterol approximately 47 mg/dL lower (135 mg/dL versus 88 mg/dL). The study was designed to run for five years, but researchers saw such dramatic declines in death and disease that they chose to cut the study short after just three years and release the results: a 36 percent reduction in heart attack risk in patients taking Lipitor compared to the control group. Plus, the risk of stroke was lowered by 27 percent in the Lipitor group. Thus, getting LDL down to ultra-low values dramatically reduces risk of heart attack and stroke.

PROSPER. This study recruited 5,804 elderly individuals, ages seventy to eighty-two, from Scotland, Ireland, and the Netherlands, all at high risk for heart disease and stroke. The patients were randomly divided into two groups: those taking Pravachol (40 mg per day) or those given a placebo. After three years, it was found that Pravachol reduced LDL cholesterol by 34 percent (from 147 mg/dL to 97 mg/dL). Furthermore, death from heart disease fell by 24 percent in the group taking Pravachol compared to the control group. This study provides further evidence supporting the notion that the lowering of heart disease risk is roughly proportional to the reduction in LDL cholesterol.

PROVE IT–TIMI-22. This trial was undertaken by Harvard researchers and was designed to compare the effects of two different statin drugs, administered at different doses, to patients drawn from eight different countries. Bristol-Myers Squibb, the maker of the older statin drug Pravachol, wanted to prove that its statin medication reduced cholesterol as well as the newer drug that had grabbed the lion's share of the market (Lipitor, manufactured by Pfizer). In this study, 4,162 patients with a recent history of heart problems were randomly assigned to take either 40 mg of Pravachol or 80 mg of Lipitor per day.

At the two-year follow-up, LDL had dropped dramatically in both groups, but to a greater extent in those taking the high dose of Lipitor (95 mg/dL versus 62 mg/dL, respectively). Regarding outcomes, it was found that 26 percent of those on Pravachol had a heart problem compared to 22 percent of those taking Lipitor and that the more intensive therapy resulted in a lower risk of death.

Thus, these five studies provide powerful evidence supporting the government's new ultra-low LDL target goal of less than 70 mg/dL (for high-risk individuals) for maximum cardio protection.

STATINS LOWER LDL

Some time ago, a group of British scientists performed three meta-analyses to answer the question "What is the effect of statins on LDL cholesterol, heart disease, and stroke?"[16] The results showed that statin drugs are highly effective medications that significantly lower LDL cholesterol levels by an average of 70 mg/dL and, by doing so, reduce the risk of a heart attack by about 60 percent and stroke by 17 percent. What's more, the researchers analyzed a number of studies that employed different methods of lowering LDL cholesterol (other than statins) and found a similar reduction in heart attack risk. This finding suggests that *the reduction in heart attack risk is attributable to the reduction in LDL cholesterol and not necessarily to the drugs themselves.* This is why the LDL-lowering combination of diet and exercise in the Cholesterol Down Plan is able to achieve LDL reduction results comparable to those of a statin drug starting dose and why the plan can be a great supplement for high-risk individuals undergoing statin treatment.

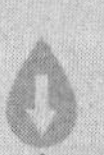

LDL: It's the End Result and Not the Means That Counts

Statins have additional healthful cardiovascular side effects beyond just LDL cholesterol reduction, termed "pleiotrophic effects." For example, statins decrease inflammation, modulate immune system response, protect against blood clots, and potentially stabilize plaque so that it is less likely to rupture and cause a heart attack. Therefore, should you take a statin drug in lieu of diet and exercise to obtain any additional cardiovascular risk reduction that these medications may possibly have to offer?

A meta-analysis showed that it is not the statin drug but the actual decrease in the LDL cholesterol number that confers these additional cardiovascular risk reductions. As such, statins do not appear to offer patients any additional risk reduction benefits beyond those observed in patients lowering LDL cholesterol via non-statin alternatives.

Sources: Jane Rutishauser, "The Role of Statins in Clinical Medicine—LDL—Cholesterol Lowering and Beyond," *Swiss Medical Weekly* 136 (2006): 41–49; Jennifer G. Robinson et al., "Pleiotrophic Effects of Statins: Benefit Beyond Cholesterol Reduction? A Meta-Regression Analysis," *Journal of the American College of Cardiology* 46 (2005): 1855–1862.

THE END OF ATHEROSCLEROSIS?

Can lowering LDL to extremely low values actually stop the progression of atherosclerosis or even promote regression of plaque? Some of the most compelling evidence to date suggesting that lower is better comes from a study of 654 people with diagnosed heart disease, termed the Reversal of Atherosclerosis with Aggressive Lipid Lowering (REVERSAL) trial.[17] Researchers randomly assigned subjects to receive either a very high dose of Lipitor (80 mg/day) or a more moderate 40 mg/day dose of Pravachol for a period of eighteen months. Results demonstrated that the high-dose Lipitor group effectively lowered LDL to an average value of 79 mg/dL (a 49 percent reduction). In contrast, the 40 mg daily dose of Pravachol resulted in a mean LDL value of 110 mg/dL (a 28 percent decline). The subjects in the high-dose Lipitor group (who attained a mean LDL of 79) showed a complete halting of the atherosclerotic process and even demonstrated a slight regression of plaque diameter compared with a slight increase in plaque size in the 40 mg Pravachol group.

The results from an international study called the ASTEROID trial (A Study to Evaluate the Effect of Rosuvastatin on Intravascular Ultrasound-Derived Coronary Atheroma Burden), involving 507 patients taking a high dose of the powerful statin drug Crestor, adds to the growing body of evidence that the lower the LDL value, the better.[18] Patients from the United States, Australia, Canada, and Europe with previously diagnosed heart disease were prescribed a daily dose of 40 mg of Crestor. After a period of two years, LDL cholesterol dropped by 53 percent and HDL cholesterol rose by 15 percent. Furthermore, researchers demonstrated an actual reversal of plaque buildup (regression) within arterial walls.

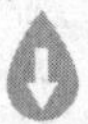

LDL Goals, LDL Values, and Risk of Heart Disease

LDL Cholesterol Level	LDL Cholesterol Category
Less than 70 mg/dL	Optimal goal for those at highest risk of heart disease
Less than 100 mg/dL	Optimal goal for most individuals
120–129 mg/dL	Near optimal/above optimal
130–159 mg/dL	Borderline high
160–189 mg/dL	High
190 mg/dL and above	Very high

Source: Alice H. Lichtenstein et al., "2021 Dietary Guidance to Improve Cardiovascular Health: A Scientific Statement from the American Heart Association," Circulation 144 (2021): e472–e487.

These data have thus established beyond a shadow of a doubt that taking aggressive measures to lower the level of LDL cholesterol saves lives. The vital message from both the established research findings and the update of the ATP III report is that *reducing LDL cholesterol to new lows halts the progression of atherosclerosis (plaque buildup) in the arteries and prevents death from cardiovascular disease.* This finding pertains to those people with high cholesterol, moderate levels, and even what was once considered low LDL cholesterol values. The latest scientific review[19] of this topic confirms the importance of LDL-C lowering in atherosclerotic cardiovascular disease prevention. Lower for longer is better!

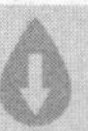

LDL: How Low Should You Go?

For the optimal prevention of heart disease, what is the ideal LDL cholesterol value to strive for? The consensus among the medical community appears to be that lower is better, especially for those at high risk for heart disease.

If you have been diagnosed with heart disease, then an LDL level of less than 70 mg/dL is a wise goal in order to halt the progression of atherosclerosis. If you are currently in good health and want to stay that way, you should aim for an LDL value of under 100 mg/dL.

HOW STATINS LOWER LDL

Statin drugs (Lipitor, Zocor, Mevacor, Crestor, Pravachol) are powerful prescription pharmaceuticals that lower circulating LDL cholesterol by inhibiting the key cholesterol-producing enzyme, HMG-CoA reductase, in the liver. Less cholesterol is produced by the liver cells, leading to an increased production of LDL receptors. More LDL receptors promote greater clearance of LDL from the bloodstream, the end result being a drop in your LDL value. And to a lesser extent, less cholesterol is packaged into VLDL, meaning less LDL is formed in the bloodstream.

Statins dramatically lower LDL levels fast. They are hailed by many in the medical world because they not only lower circulating LDL levels but also significantly lessen the inflammatory response within the arterial wall (as evidenced by a decline in the level of C-reactive protein). Ultimately, statin drugs save lives. They are considered by many in the medical establishment to be the wonder drugs of the twenty-first century.

STATINS SAVE LIVES, BUT ARE THEY SAFE?

"My doctor has me on a low-dose statin, but my LDL just won't go down to where she wants it. She would like me to up my dosage, but I am afraid of the terrible side effects I have been reading about."

Several of my patients have expressed concern not only with the potential for serious side effects but also with the safety of America's supply of prescription drugs in general. Statins are the first-choice drug for patients at high risk of cardiovascular disease and are used safely by millions of people around the world. However, as with any prescription medication, there are side effects; in rare instances they can be serious and even fatal. Here are some statin facts you may not be aware of.

- The majority of LDL cholesterol lowering occurs with the lowest statin dosages (10 mg). Up the dose and you get diminishing returns. Doubling the statin dosage results in only an additional 5–6 percent drop in LDL cholesterol.[20] Another good reason to question upping your dose of statins is that taking a higher dose significantly increases the potential for side effects.
- All statins have some risk associated with them. Just how much risk? Case in point: the recent rash of bad press surrounding Crestor, the strongest member of the statin family, has caused much anxiety. High doses of Crestor have resulted in reports of a rare and potentially fatal muscle disorder, known as rhabdomyolysis, that can cause kidney failure. Asian Americans, in particular, were found to be at increased risk for severe complications from higher doses of Crestor. What's more, another cholesterol-lowering drug, Baycol, was voluntarily pulled from the market more than twenty years ago after it was linked to at least thirty-one deaths.

- The fear of side effects from statin drug therapy should be put into perspective with the understanding that the higher the dose, the greater the likelihood of side effects. Combining a statin drug with a fibrate, another type of cholesterol-lowering drug (specifically a fibrate called Lopid), is not advised because the combination is more likely to produce side effects than statins taken alone. Combining statins with niacin, another treatment option for lowering cholesterol, has also been associated with some evidence of liver problems.
- The use of statins in conjunction with a therapeutic lifestyle plan, such as Cholesterol Down, is an effective alternative to upping your statin dose.

WHAT ARE POSSIBLE SIDE EFFECTS TO WATCH FOR?

"My doctor put me on Lipitor, but I just couldn't take the side effects—I felt nauseous, and my muscles ached. Is there any way I can lower my cholesterol without taking prescription drugs?"

Many of my patients have confided in me that they cannot tolerate the side effects from even the lowest-dose statin drug treatment but are concerned because their physician has recommended medication to reduce an unhealthy cholesterol level. Side effects of taking statin drugs can include headache, gastrointestinal problems, fatigue, flu-like symptoms, and myalgia (characterized by muscle weakness or unusual muscular aches and pains generally not associated with the breakdown of muscle tissue).[21] Liver problems (detected by an abnormal increase in liver enzymes released into the bloodstream) or severe muscle problems such as myopathy and rhabdomyolysis are rare, but these potentially serious side effects have been recorded in statin therapy patients.

Myopathy occurs when muscular weakness, aches, and pains are accompanied by significant and measurable muscle tissue breakdown. Rhabdomyolysis is when muscle involvement is so severe that the breakdown products saturate the bloodstream (as evidenced by myoglobin, a muscle protein, coloring the urine brown) and can progress to a life-threatening situation such as kidney failure.

Another potential cause for concern is the marked decrease in the blood of a compound called coenzyme Q_{10} (CoQ_{10}), which has been observed in patients taking statin drugs. CoQ_{10} (aka ubiquinone) is found in large concentration in the energy-producing powerhouses of the cell, the mitochondria. A large amount of CoQ_{10} is located in the cells of the heart muscle. CoQ_{10} functions as a key player in transforming the energy from the food we eat into chemical energy known as adenosine triphosphate. Furthermore, CoQ_{10} has antioxidant properties that can help prevent the oxidation of LDL cholesterol.

Some scientists believe that the depletion of CoQ_{10} by statin drugs contributes to the occurrence of many of the adverse side effects discussed above. In fact, Canada requires that all statin drugs carry a warning label alerting consumers that the drugs deplete CoQ_{10} levels in the blood. Research has surfaced that bolsters the notion that statin drugs deplete cellular CoQ_{10} levels. Researchers at Columbia University's College of Physicians and Surgeons measured CoQ_{10} levels in thirty-four patients before and after placing them on a high dose of Lipitor (80 mg/day) for a period of thirty days.[22] There was a marked decrease in the blood concentration of CoQ_{10} after thirty days of treatment, with the average blood level dropping by half. The researchers concluded that the depletion of CoQ_{10} could help explain the most common negative side effects associated with statin use.

On May 24, 2002, Julian Whitaker, M.D., filed a citizen's petition to the U.S. Food and Drug Administration to change the statin labels so that they are required to mention that HMG-CoA reductase inhibitors (statins) block the synthesis of CoQ_{10}, which may have deleterious side effects. He suggests that all patients be encouraged to take CoQ_{10} supplements, which are very safe.[23] Unfortunately, not all scientists agree. A recent double-blind, randomized clinical trial on the effect of CoQ_{10} supplementation on statin-induced myalgia showed no effect.[24] Despite these results, I still recommend taking a CoQ_{10} supplement if you are taking statin medication.

The Bottom Line on Statins

Statin drugs are generally safe and have become the essential treatment for those at high risk for heart disease. High doses cut LDL to ultra-low values, yet you must heed the caveat: high dosages increase the risk of serious side effects. There is a solution to this problem. The goal should be to get LDL to target levels, using the lowest dose possible. If a high-dose statin is advocated but you are wary of or cannot tolerate taking the higher dosage, consider adding in a more natural strategy. The Cholesterol Down Plan, combined with your lower-dose statin drug, may be the perfect means to help you reach your LDL goal.

STATINS ALONE ARE NOT ENOUGH

"My doctor has me on a statin pill. My cholesterol dropped from 290 to 180 mg/dL, so I can pretty much eat whatever I want." This particular middle-aged male patient has a strong family history (both parents died of heart disease), experienced overweight (with the fat concentrated around his belly—a dangerous location), doesn't exercise, and eats a heavy meat-based, high-fat, low-fiber diet. My guess is that the statin drugs will not fully protect him against succumbing to heart disease before his time, despite the significant drop in his cholesterol level. I see this quite often and call it the "statin mentality." It is human nature to look for a quick fix, a Band-Aid approach that salves the guilt and allows for continuation of an unhealthy lifestyle, masking the reality of the situation. Don't fool yourself into thinking that taking a daily statin pill will reverse the effects of the atherosclerosis-inducing lifestyle that is all too typical among Americans. How many times do you order a thick slab of prime rib, a baked potato smothered in butter, and a gargantuan slice of New York–style cheesecake and think, "I better take my Lipitor with my coffee"? This type of behavior is not exactly heart-healthy. In this regard, statins are not a cure-all, and their LDL-lowering effects may be overwhelmed by multiple heart disease risk factors and unhealthy lifestyle practices such as lack of exercise, a propensity for weight gain (especially around the middle), and/or a low-fiber diet full of saturated fat and cholesterol. The Cholesterol Down Plan not only helps you fight high cholesterol but also provides a diet and exercise prescription that either in combination with statin treatment or on its own helps lower these other risk factors for cardiovascular disease as well.

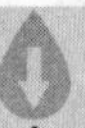

Lower for Longer Is Better

The risk of a heart attack is closely correlated with the cumulative exposure to LDL cholesterol, the key driver of atherosclerotic heart disease. This means that your risk significantly increases depending on the magnitude of your LDL level multiplied by the years of exposure. Scientists have proven that to prevent heart disease, lower for longer is better. The ideal preventive treatment is to apply a combination of therapies to achieve a robust and sustained reduction in LDL. If you are concerned about the effects of significantly lowering LDL, research has proven that achieving very low LDLC is both feasible and safe.

Source: Omar Mhaimeed et al., "The Importance of LDL-C Lowering in Atherosclerotic Cardiovascular Disease Prevention: Lower for Longer Is Better," *American Journal of Preventive Cardiology* 18 (June 2024): 100649, https://doi.org/10.1016/j.ajpc.2024.100649.

DIET—NOT DRUGS—SHOULD BE THE *FIRST* LINE OF DEFENSE

What do you do if you've tried statins to lower your high LDL cholesterol but with adverse consequences? What if you're distrustful of taking prescription drugs in general? After decades of drug recalls and ongoing concerns about statin side effects—from muscle pain to cognitive issues—a cautious public rightly questions whether the pharmaceutical route is their only option, and Americans are increasingly seeking healthier, drug-free alternatives for managing cholesterol.

The NCEP continues to play a role in promoting healthy heart awareness and providing guidance related to cholesterol management. While the specific recommendations and approaches have evolved over time, the NCEP remains a key resource in the field of cardiovascular health. The truth is that statins should not be the first line of defense against high cholesterol. Doctors were instructed by ATP III to first initiate "therapeutic lifestyle change"—namely, diet and exercise—if their patient's LDL is above the desired goal. If diet and exercise alone fail, only then should doctors consider drug therapy.[25] In fact, the government's NCEP report continues to emphasize the importance of therapeutic lifestyle change (a heart-healthy diet, such as the Cholesterol Down Plan, employing proven cholesterol-lowering foods and exercise in addition to weight management) as the cornerstone for cholesterol management.

Several of the dietary steps in the Cholesterol Down Plan work in a drug-like fashion, almost the dietary equivalent of taking a statin, a bile acid sequestrant (such as Welchol), and a cholesterol absorption blocker (such as Zetia). Take this more natural lifestyle approach and watch your LDL plummet—without the side effects!

CHAPTER 3

Cholesterol Down: A Combination Therapy as Effective as Statins

The combination approach of nine foods plus exercise in the Cholesterol Down Plan developed out of my own approach to naturally reducing my LDL cholesterol. My success with the plan, as well as my patients' success, provided proof that the complementary, combined effect of several simple diet and lifestyle manipulations is extremely effective in lowering LDL cholesterol levels—far more than a single food or exercise. This is because each component lowers LDL to a different degree, and each involves a somewhat different mechanism of action.

ORIGIN OF NATURAL COMBINATION THERAPY: PORTFOLIO DIET

In 2002, a group of Canadian scientists at the University of Toronto originated the concept of combining several previously established solitary LDL-lowering dietary strategies into a single treatment, which they called the Dietary Portfolio Approach to Cholesterol Reduction. The scientists tested this novel protocol for the first time in people with high cholesterol and achieved miraculous results—a 29 percent drop in LDL levels. Volunteers in the Canadian study were placed on the combination Portfolio diet containing soy foods, plant sterols (plant chemicals that block cholesterol absorption), soluble fiber (from oats, barley, legumes, eggplant, okra, and Metamucil), and almonds.[1] After four weeks, LDL cholesterol fell an astounding 29 percent in the Portfolio diet group, the same LDL reduction observed in the subjects adhering to a standard low-fat diet and taking the statin drug Mevacor. The researchers concluded that the dramatic reduction in LDL cholesterol from the Portfolio diet was comparable to the LDL-lowering results seen with a starting dose of a prescription statin medication.

Diet Works as Well as Statins in Lowering LDL Cholesterol

Would the LDL-lowering power of the Portfolio diet rival that of a starting dose of a cholesterol-lowering statin drug? The answer is a resounding yes. The same Canadian researchers who originated the Portfolio diet performed a study directly comparing the Portfolio diet with a statin drug in subjects with high LDL cholesterol.[2] After just four weeks, both groups lowered their LDL to the same extent, by approximately 30 percent. This exciting discovery demonstrates that the simple daily combination of foods with known cholesterol-lowering effects can be just as powerful as a starting dose of a statin drug in reducing the level of "bad" cholesterol.

ADDITIONAL SCIENTIFIC SUPPORT FOR THE EFFICACY OF NATURAL COMBINATION THERAPY

Another study investigating the synergy of two dietary steps together found that a daily combination of oats and plant sterols exhibits a powerful cholesterol-lowering effect. A 2003 study published in the *Journal of Nutrition* showed that a daily combination of 2.8 grams of beta-glucan (primarily from oats) and 1.8 grams of phytosterols (concurrent with a low-fat NCEP Step 1 diet) was able to reduce LDL cholesterol by an additional 8 percent over the negligible 1 percent drop seen with the traditional Step 1 diet alone.[3] Additional findings out of Stanford

University provide added support for the notion that combining several foods has a dramatic impact on LDL cholesterol.[4] Researchers compared the LDL-reducing power of a traditional low-fat diet with a plant-based low-fat diet. Adding in a daily dose of soy protein (16 grams) and garlic (1½ cloves) to the plant-based low-fat diet rich in whole grains, beans, fruit, vegetables, legumes, nuts, and seeds lowered subjects' LDL cholesterol by approximately 9 percent in just four weeks. That amount was more than double the conventional low-fat diet's LDL cholesterol-lowering potential.

The Results Are In: A Portfolio-Style Diet Proven to Lower the Risk of Heart Disease

The proof is in the scientific pudding. Three large studies following over 120,000 men and women over thirty years have recently proven that long-term adherence to a Portfolio-style diet filled with plant protein (from foods such as legumes), nuts and seeds, soluble fiber sources (soluble fiber forms a gel-like substance when mixed with water and can be found in many foods, including oats, apples, and chia seeds), phytosterols and plant monounsaturated fat produces significant heart health benefits. People who ate a Portfolio-style diet significantly cut their risk of heart disease and stroke, exhibited a much more favorable LDL profile, and had less inflammation (a driver of atherosclerosis) compared to people who did not eat this way.

Source: Andrea J. Glenn et al., "Portfolio Diet Score and Risk of Cardiovascular Disease: Findings from 3 Prospective Cohort Studies," *Circulation* 148 (2023): 1750–1763.

Need more recent evidence that the power of the Cholesterol Down suggested steps, combined, dramatically lower LDL cholesterol? A double-blind randomized clinical trial[5] studied the effects of snacks containing a compendium of cholesterol-lowering bioactive food compounds (fiber and phytosterols) on fasting LDL cholesterol in eighteen subjects unwilling to take a statin drug. The results? After just four weeks, the subjects' LDL cholesterol dropped an average of 9 mg/dL.

LIVE LONGER AND PREVENT HEART PROBLEMS: THE EUROPEAN "POLYMEAL" STRATEGY

There's no shortage of proof that natural combination therapy—the safe, non-pharmacological alternative for slashing cholesterol—works. Another combination strategy of special heart-healthy foods, this time concocted by European scientists whose findings were published in the prestigious *British Medical Journal,* is called the "polymeal."[6] The daily polymeal diet includes six types of foods:

- Red wine (5 ounces, or 150 milliliters)
- Fish (4 ounces, or 114 grams)
- Dark chocolate (3.5 ounces, or 100 grams)
- Fruits and vegetables (14 ounces, or 400 grams)
- Garlic (0.1 ounces, or 2.7 grams)
- Almonds (2.4 ounces, or 68 grams)

The scientists calculated that eating a daily combination of all these foods could theoretically reduce the risk of cardiovascular disease by a spectacular 76 percent. Life expectancy could be prolonged 4.8 years in women and 6.6 years in men and heart problems delayed 8.1 years in women and 9 years in men.

THE CHOLESTEROL DOWN PLAN

These other diets laid the foundation for the potent combination therapy model I used to develop the Cholesterol Down Plan. Cholesterol Down takes nine individually active cholesterol-lowering food ingredients—all scientifically shown to independently reduce LDL cholesterol—and combines them on a daily basis with a scientifically proven LDL-lowering exercise program.[7] In effect, the simple concept of *combining all these proven cholesterol-lowering foods with an exercise routine is as effective as combining several types of cholesterol-lowering drugs.* All the ingredients are available at your local supermarket and are no more dangerous or expensive than almonds, oatmeal, or an apple. The result is a highly effective, easy-to-follow plan that reduces LDL cholesterol as much as cholesterol-lowering prescription drugs, but without the side effects.

Each of the steps of the Cholesterol Down Plan lowers "bad" cholesterol in a slightly different way. In this manner, the combination approach provides substantially more cholesterol-lowering strength than a single therapeutic treatment. Plant sterols, for example (see Chapter 10), work through a different mechanism than soy protein (see Chapter 11). Whereas sterols lower cholesterol by blocking absorption from the intestine, soy protein lowers cholesterol by increasing LDL receptors on the liver, resulting in increased LDL cholesterol removal from the bloodstream. Daily doses of both soy and plant sterols work jointly to cut cholesterol much more than either in isolation. This approach is similar to combining a statin drug (which reduces cholesterol production in the liver and increases LDL clearance from the blood) with another drug such as Zetia (which blocks cholesterol absorption from the intestine). In this way, all ten steps of the Cholesterol Down Plan work together to pack a very powerful punch in lowering LDL levels by up to 47 percent, comparable to the effectiveness of statin drugs but without the side effects.

DAILY CHECKLIST MAKES PLAN EASY TO FOLLOW

I encourage my patients to use the Ten-Step Daily Checklist located in Appendix 1. Think of all ten steps as the equivalent to the daily statin dose—it's therefore essential to get them all in.

The next ten chapters provide a set of simple, healthful food and exercise prescriptions that give safe and measurable cholesterol-lowering results in as little as four weeks' time. Read on to begin with Step 1 of the daily checklist and start to get your cholesterol down!

PART II

The Ten-Step Cholesterol Down Plan

CHAPTER 4

Step 1: Eat Oatmeal

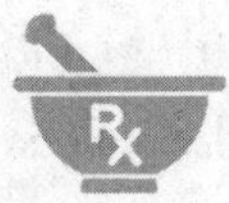

Eat 1 cup of oatmeal every day (most therapeutic dose: 3 grams of beta-glucan per day).

THE WHOLE-GRAIN GOODNESS OF OATMEAL

A patient once said to me, "My grandfather ate oatmeal every morning of his life and he lived to be a hundred." My response was, "Do what your grandfather did."

Whole-grain oats are tasty and inexpensive and have a long history of health benefits. This simple grain has been shown to lower cholesterol and blood pressure, normalize blood sugar, appease the appetite, and ameliorate intestinal problems. Remember the oat bran craze of the 1980s? That phenomenon grew out of an overwhelming amount of scientific evidence that began to build during the 1960s, linking oat consumption with dramatic declines in blood cholesterol. The FDA recommends consuming more than 3 grams of oat beta-glucan each day to enjoy its beneficial heart health effects.

WHAT MAKES A GRAIN WHOLE?

Whole grains are kernels of grain that are consumed with all three naturally occurring components still intact: the outer fiber-rich bran layer, the middle energy-packed endosperm, and the inner nutrient-rich germ layer. The outer bran holds the mineral cache, with up to 80 percent of all the minerals found in the kernel concentrated in this coating. The bran also contains fiber, protein, and some B vitamins. The endosperm is a pocket of energy-yielding starch (complex carbohydrate), some protein, iron, and a minuscule amount of B vitamins, all used to nourish the growing seedling. The germ is packed with a gold mine of vitamins including vitamin E (wheat germ is one of the richest sources of vitamin E), B vitamins (especially high in folate), some trace minerals (iron, magnesium, selenium, and potassium), fiber, and phytosterols (plant hormones that lower cholesterol).

Debby's Story

Debby G., age fifty-four

Pre: Total cholesterol: 245 mg/dL; LDL cholesterol: 147 mg/dL

Post: Total cholesterol: 206 mg/dL; LDL cholesterol: 106 mg/dL

28 percent reduction in LDL cholesterol

Debby exhibited a classic case of statin intolerance. A middle-aged woman in excellent physical condition with a lifetime of healthy eating habits under her belt, she was surprised that her cholesterol had become dangerously high. Her physician placed her on a statin drug, and within a few weeks she began to experience unpleasant side effects. Her doctor switched her to another statin drug, but her side effects worsened. She shares her experience here.

I am my mother's child from looks to stature—we even have the same voice. Mom has been on cholesterol meds for many years. Even before I discovered I had high cholesterol, I was wary of taking cholesterol medication, as I witnessed her frequent complaints about aches, pains, and stomach problems from the cholesterol meds. I haven't eaten red meat in thirty years, chicken in twenty, and have always watched my intake of fats and sweets. I exercise at least five days a week. When my physician insisted I start statins, I shuddered, despite the fact that my cholesterol was so high. Within a few weeks, my toes, fingers, and knees hurt so badly I couldn't exercise. I went off the treatment for a few weeks until the doctor insisted I go on another statin. I started taking Lescol, and within a few weeks the same thing happened again, only worse. Now I couldn't even walk down the steps in my house. I immediately went in for a blood test and that same day received a call to stop the drug ASAP. It was affecting my liver.

After some time, my cholesterol spiked to 286. My doctor insisted I take a cholesterol absorption blocker called Zetia. I was able to get my cholesterol down in three months to 244. "That's as good as it's going to get," I thought—until I met with Dr. Janet Brill and decided to follow her program for three months. After just four weeks, my total cholesterol went down to 206 (and my "bad" cholesterol dropped from 142 to 106). Her diet is a great routine. I have never been hungry! The soy has eased my hot flashes, and I don't need to take my medication for acid reflux as often. This is a routine I will easily continue with for the rest of my life.

WHY WHOLE GRAINS ARE BEST

When grains are milled or refined, they are stripped of the outer bran and germ layers and thus lose many of the naturally occurring vitamins and minerals, healthful fats, and phytonutrients. Processing leaves behind only the starchy endosperm. In 1942 the U.S. government passed a law requiring iron and B vitamin enrichment of processed grains to combat vitamin deficiency as a result of eating refined products, devoid of their natural lode of vitamins and minerals. This is why when you purchase a refined grain product such as white bread or white rice (made solely from the endosperm of grains), it will by law be "enriched," meaning a few nutrients have been added back—often niacin, iron, thiamin, riboflavin, and folate. Unfortunately, what is lost in the processing and not required to be replaced are wholesome nutrients such as fiber, vitamin E, several B vitamins, potassium, minerals such as manganese, magnesium, copper, and zinc, and various healthful phytochemicals such as lignans, flavonoids, and saponins. Clearly, whole grains are the far superior choice over refined grains for fiber, vitamins, minerals, and other important nutrients.

WHOLE GRAINS FOR GOOD HEALTH

A diet rich in whole grains—rather than highly processed, refined grains—has been linked with reduced risk of heart disease, stroke, type 2 diabetes, obesity, and certain types of cancers, as well as with lower blood pressure and improved bowel function.

The connection between whole grains and heart health is where the science is particularly strong, with a huge body of research backing the notion that diets high in whole grains reduce your risk for heart disease. Data from the Iowa Women's Health Study have provided sound evidence that whole grains keep a woman's cardiovascular system in good health, even after menopause.[1] Researchers took detailed dietary and health histories from 34,492 postmenopausal women between the ages of fifty-five and sixty-nine and followed them over a nine-year period. The women who consumed the most servings of whole grains had more than a 30 percent decrease in risk of death from heart disease than the women who ate less than one serving per day.

Whole grains also stop inflammation of the arteries, according to a study published in the *Journal of Nutrition.*[2] Inflammation is related to plaque buildup, or atherosclerosis. C-reactive protein is a protein circulating in the bloodstream that is used by doctors as a marker for inflammation and a predictor of future cardiovascular disease (a value above 3 mg/L is considered indicative of high risk for heart disease). Analyses of almost 4,000 American men and women showed that the higher the fiber intake (whole grains are one of the best sources of dietary fiber), the lower the blood concentration of C-reactive protein.

What's good for the heart is also good for the brain, according to a study by researchers at Harvard Medical School.[3] As part of the famed Nurses' Health Study, 75,521 women nurses between the ages of thirty-eight and sixty-three were followed for ten years, providing dietary and health data at four separate intervals. The study found that nurses who ate two to three servings of whole grains daily were 43 percent less likely to have an ischemic stroke (blockage of the artery feeding the brain) than those women eating less than one serving per day.

The benefits of whole grains are not just for women—eating whole grains helps men live longer and healthier lives, too. Boston researchers examined associations between whole-grain cereal intake and risk of death from all causes in data drawn from 86,190 U.S. male physicians participating in the Physicians' Health Study. Researchers followed the physicians over a period averaging five and a half years.[4] Higher whole-grain cereal consumption compared to refined grains was found to significantly reduce the risk of dying not only from heart disease but in fact from all causes.

HOW MUCH WHOLE-GRAIN FOOD SHOULD YOU EAT?

The USDA Dietary Guidelines for Americans 2020–2025 (www.dietaryguidelines.gov) recommends that at least half of total grains consumed should be whole grains. If you're like most Americans, though, your whole-grain intake is woefully short of this goal. According to the USDA, on average, 98 percent of us fall below recommendations for whole grains. The reason, say some nutrition scientists, is that many Americans have opted not to cook and eat whole grains because they take longer to cook, chew, and digest than refined grains. Perhaps it is also true that outside of your grocery or health food store, whole grains are nearly impossible to find. When was the last time you ordered quinoa at McDonald's?

My advice is that you don't follow the path of the over 40 percent of all adults who eat no whole grains at all. Instead, try to get in at least three servings each day to increase your fiber and nutrient intake and begin reaping the plethora of health benefits. Eating a morning bowl of oatmeal is a great first step to get you a third of the way there.

THE CHOLESTEROL-LOWERING POWER OF OATS

Decades of research, including more than fifty clinical trials, have consistently demonstrated that oats lower cholesterol, particularly LDL cholesterol.[5] Furthermore, oats reduce LDL cholesterol without a concurrent reduction in the level of "good" HDL cholesterol—and may even raise HDL. Some time ago, researchers at the University of California, Davis, performed a study in which 84 grams (roughly 3 ounces) of oat bran (the most soluble-fiber-rich portion of oats) were added to the subjects' usual low-fat diet. LDL cholesterol fell an amazing 17 percent in just six weeks.[6]

Why should you choose oatmeal over a refined wheat cereal such as Special K for breakfast? Researchers at Colorado State University showed that eating oats can change the characteristics of LDL particles to a more desirable fatter and fluffier shape.[7] Thirty-six subjects were given either an oat cereal or a wheat cereal for twelve weeks. Not only did the amount of dangerous small and dense LDL particles drop considerably in the oat-eating group, but members also showed beneficially altered LDL particle size. This change protects you against heart disease because the smaller or denser LDL particles are more susceptible to oxidation, have less of an affinity for the liver LDL receptors (recall that the receptors are the only way out of the bloodstream for LDL), remain in the bloodstream longer than larger LDL particles, and can slip into the arterial wall easier.

BETA-GLUCAN: THE KEY INGREDIENT

What makes oats truly a cholesterol-lowering wonder food is a special ingredient within the grain, a type of soluble fiber called beta-glucan. There are two types of fiber found in plants, water-soluble fiber and insoluble fiber. Oats contain both types and are an especially rich source of the soluble type, particularly beta-glucan.

Beta-glucan consists of a string of glucose molecules that the human body is not equipped to break apart or digest. In terms of lowering LDL cholesterol, this string acts like an intestinal sponge, soaking up the excess and driving it out of the body. A number of studies show that the more beta-glucan consumed, the greater the drop in LDL cholesterol. A recent meta-analysis of thirteen randomized controlled trials appraising the effect of regular oat beta-glucan intake on lipid profiles indicated that oat beta-glucan significantly lowers LDL cholesterol.[8]

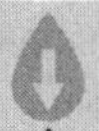

Beta-Glucan In Oats Drains LDL

Randomized clinical trials provide the highest level of evidence to establish cause and effect in clinical research. A meta-analysis is a powerful statistical tool for combining the findings of such trials. As mentioned above, a recent meta-analysis of thirteen trials with close to 1,000 participants found that only those individuals consuming oat beta-glucan daily exhibited significant declines in their LDL cholesterol values at the end of the trial period. The authors state that oats most likely cause LDL to decrease due to the ability of beta-glucan to enhance bile acid excretion, which helps our bodies metabolize and eliminate cholesterol.

Source: J. Yu et al., "Effects of Oat Beta-Glucan Intake on Lipid Profiles in Hypercholesterolemic Adults: A Systematic Review and Meta-Analysis of Randomized Controlled Trials," *Nutrients* 14, no. 10 (2022): 2043. https://doi.org/10.3390/nu14102043.

HOW DOES BETA-GLUCAN SLASH LDL CHOLESTEROL?

Beta-glucan attacks LDL by several different methods acting in concert.

Method of Attack #1. The main cholesterol-lowering method is beta-glucan's previously mentioned ability to transform itself into a viscous, gel-like sponge. The string of glucose molecules forms a mass of jelly-like fiber, which absorbs bile juice from the intestines and reduces the speed at which food and waste move through and exit them. Recall that bile juice is formed in the liver and contains large amounts of cholesterol and bile acids (formerly cholesterol). Bile acids are typically recycled back from the lower intestine to the liver. But with beta-glucan consumption, bile acids are diverted, absorbed within the beta-glucan mass, and excreted. How does beta-glucan sequester the bile? Both the high solubility in water and the viscous nature of beta-glucan play a key role in this fiber's ability to lower cholesterol. *Viscosity* refers to the capacity of binding, and this particular fiber can bind an extraordinary amount, up to 200 times its weight in water. Only highly soluble, viscous fibers are able to form the sticky substance that works like glue to bind the intestinal contents for excretion.

Therefore, the primary mechanism beta-glucan uses to lower LDL is increasing the excretion of bile acids. This is precisely how prescription cholesterol-lowering drugs called bile acid sequestrants (such as Questran) work.[9] With the increased excretion of bile acids, reabsorption is thus reduced and the liver is deprived of its normal return flow. Fewer bile acids returning to the liver via the normal recycling route mean that the liver cells are prompted to make more bile acids (from cholesterol) to match the excretion rate and replenish the depleted bile acids. The result? The liver is forced to grab the circulating LDL in the bloodstream to restock the cholesterol supply, causing the blood LDL cholesterol level to drop.

Method of Attack #2. A second mechanism by which beta-glucan lowers LDL cholesterol relates to the bulky nature of foods high in beta-glucan and the effect this has as food moves down the intestine. The viscosity of the intestinal contents and the sheer bulk of the stool thicken what's called the unstirred water layer, the river of water that is next to the cells lining the intestine. This water layer is a barrier that must be penetrated by the cholesterol transporter known as a micelle before cholesterol can get to the second transporter, the protein channel called NPC 1L1, for passage into the cells lining the upper intestine. Soluble fiber thickens the water layer, making it more resistant to penetration by the micelle and thus thwarting absorption of cholesterol. The cholesterol, therefore, never makes it to the NPC 1L1 transporter that would have provided passage inside the intestinal cell layer. Micelle formation is also impaired. The result of both of these scenarios is less cholesterol absorbed from the intestinal pool and packaged into big balls of fat known as chylomicrons. Therefore, the chylomicrons returning to the liver have only a partial supply of cholesterol, meaning less cholesterol to be packaged and re-secreted from the liver as VLDL. The end result of all this is less LDL circulating in the blood.

Method of Attack #3. Beta-glucan slows the rate of glucose (sugar) absorption into the body. Less sugar in the blood means less insulin is released from the pancreas. Insulin increases production of cholesterol by liver cells, so less insulin translates into less cholesterol produced.

Method of Attack #4. Fermentation of beta-glucan in the large intestine by friendly bacteria results in the formation of short-chain fatty acids: acetate, butyrate, and propionate. These fatty acids, propionate in particular, are absorbed in the colon, travel to the liver, and interfere with the main enzyme involved in cholesterol production, HMG-CoA reductase.[10] If this scenario looks familiar, it should. This is the same mechanism that statin drugs use to quell the liver cells' internal production of cholesterol.

Method of Attack #5. The composition of the oat kernel, namely, its unusual amino acid profile and high antioxidant content, serves to reduce LDL cholesterol in varying ways (discussed in greater depth later in this chapter).

HOW MUCH BETA-GLUCAN DOES IT TAKE TO LOWER LDL CHOLESTEROL?

Current dietary guidelines recommend increasing soluble fiber intake, including beta-glucan, to help lower cholesterol. While the FDA recommends 28 grams of total fiber daily for a 2,000-calorie diet, experts suggest that 5–10 grams of this should be soluble fiber for optimal cholesterol-lowering benefits.[11] A more specific recommendation from the FDA specifies that you consume 3 grams of beta-glucan daily to lower LDL cholesterol. This was based on a meta-analysis—the results of numerous studies analyzed all together to come up with a main conclusion—of nineteen studies.[12] Therefore, including 3 grams of beta-glucan (the amount found in a bowl of oatmeal for breakfast) will meet the FDA's daily goal, help fulfill the NCEP recommendation, and truly start your day off right.

HOW ANTIOXIDANTS PROTECT YOUR ARTERIES

Oats contain an array of powerful antioxidants, warriors in the fight against rogue free radicals that harm healthy cells and cause the oxidation of LDL, the first step in the cascade of events leading to plaque formation. Antioxidants can fight off this oxidative stress as well as decrease inflammation, two key factors in the process of atherosclerosis. Oats are noteworthy among grains because they contain an extraordinary type of antioxidant called avenanthramides, unique to oats and particularly instrumental in fighting LDL corrosion.

Should You Just Eat Oat Bran Instead of Oatmeal?

Oat bran, the outer layer of the grain, is the most concentrated source of beta-glucan and is also home to a powerful type of antioxidant found only in oats. There are, however, highly nutritious components found in the two other parts of the oat kernel—the germ and the endosperm—that you would not benefit from if you routinely chose to eat just the bran. For example, the potent antioxidant vitamin E compounds (tocopherols and tocotrienols) are located in the germ and endosperm. In fact, there is some evidence that tocotrienols reduce LDL cholesterol by interfering with the main cholesterol-manufacturing enzyme HMG-CoA reductase. Eat just the bran and you miss out on this potential LDL-cutting nutrient. I recommend that you eat whole oat products and add in some extra oat bran. That way you get the extra beta-glucan and all the other nutrients found in the germ and endosperm, too.

Sources: David M. Petersen, "Oat Tocols: Concentration and Stability in Oat Products and Distribution Within the Kernel," *Cereal Chemistry* 72, no. 1 (1995): 21–24; Asaf A. Qureshi et al., "The Structure of an Inhibitor of Cholesterol Biosynthesis Isolated from Barley," *Journal of Biological Chemistry* 261, no. 23 (1986): 10544–10550.

Nutritionists at the Jean Mayer USDA Human Nutrition Research Center on Aging at Tufts University recently provided scientific evidence about how this particular antioxidant enhances resistance of human LDL particles to oxidation (free radical damage).[13] LDL was collected from human volunteers and exposed to copper (a mineral that binds to LDL and degrades it) in the lab. The unique combination of antioxidants found in oats, including avenanthramides, were able to fend off LDL breakdown for an extended period of time. The higher the amount of antioxidant, the greater the amount of time before LDL became oxidized.

Another study at Tufts University demonstrated the ability of this same oat antioxidant to decrease the inflammatory response that so heavily contributes to atherosclerosis.[14] In the experiment, scientists isolated the avenanthramides (found in highest concentration in the outer bran layer of the oat grain), purified them, and exposed them to human aorta arterial wall cells for a twenty-four-hour period. After incubation, observations revealed significantly fewer adhesion molecules surfacing on the inner arterial wall (adhesion molecules are indicative of an inflammatory reaction) and also fewer blood cells sticking to the walls. The sticking of blood cells to artery walls via adhesion molecules is a key step in the atherosclerotic process. Thus, oat antioxidants have a unique two-pronged protective effect: the strong antioxidant power of avenanthramides fights LDL corrosion (a major step in atherosclerosis), and the anti-inflammatory power of the antioxidant mix interferes with the ability of blood cells to stick to arterial walls, a key process associated with plaque formation.

AMINO ACIDS REDUCE YOUR RISK FOR HEART ATTACK

Oats have a unique amino acid ratio that contributes to their ability to promote heart health. Specifically, oats contain a larger proportion of the amino acid arginine relative to the amount of the amino acid lysine, and arginine is believed to decrease the production of LDL cholesterol and increase its breakdown.[15]

The amino acid arginine is a precursor for a substance called nitric oxide, a potent blood vessel relaxant and a key factor in arginine's well-known ability to lower blood pressure. Arginine has also been shown to lessen the blood's ability to clot by decreasing platelet stickiness. This anti-clotting mechanism could theoretically reduce your chances of succumbing to a heart attack, as a blood clot sealing off the vessel is the last and often fatal step in the series of events leading to a heart attack. Arginine is also considered an immune system booster and is often given to severely immune-compromised individuals, such as those with AIDS, or to reduce postoperative infections.

OATMEAL HELPS WITH WEIGHT LOSS

There's another great reason to order oatmeal instead of cornflakes for breakfast at your local diner. Whole-grain oats are packed with nutrients and are much higher in fiber than their refined wheat cousins. The fiber helps keep you full and in doing so regulates your appetite. Studies show that beta-glucan increases the amount of a hormone (cholecystokinin) released into the intestine that makes you feel full. Also, the beta-glucan in oats delays gastric emptying, which would contribute to increased satiety. Whole grains take longer to chew than refined grains, giving the brain more time to get that signal from the stomach that food has arrived. Oats are loaded with protein, containing the most protein of all the grains commonly eaten in the United States—twice the amount found in a kernel of brown rice.

Of all the macronutrients (carbs, fat, and protein), protein is the most filling. Moreover, not only are oats good for taking the edge off your appetite, but they can also help with fat loss by lowering the blood sugar and insulin response after eating. Because insulin is a hormone that promotes fat storage, reducing the amount released by the pancreas following a meal could aid in your weight loss endeavors.

As previously mentioned, weight is a factor leading to cardiovascular disease, and living with overweight can contribute to increased levels of LDL cholesterol. Weight control, therefore, is an important added benefit of eating oatmeal.

WHICH VARIETY OF OATS IS THE HEALTHIEST?

Eat your oats! Oatmeal is a whole grain regardless of whether it is instant, old-fashioned, or quick-cooking. The difference lies in how finely the grain has been ground and thus how fast it cooks. There are all kinds of oats on the market. Read on and become an oat connoisseur.

GROATS

The whole oat kernels that have been hulled (the inedible chaff has been removed), cleaned, and conditioned right off the farm are called oat groats, the least processed of all the oats on the market and, therefore, the ones that retain all the natural nutrients. Oat groats are typically found only in health food or specialty stores. Goldilocks and the rest of us recognize oat groats as porridge, the name given in Europe to cooked oat groats. Porridge also is a traditional Scottish breakfast and is made by simply cooking the groats for an extended period of time; porridge is typically cooked for about an hour and a half on the stovetop. Oat groats are the most nutritious form of oats but are chewy and need to be cooked a very long time.

STEEL-CUT OATS

Another type of oat kernel is steel-cut oats (also called Scotch oats or Irish oatmeal). After harvest from the field, cleaning, hulling, and conditioning, steel-cut oats are then chopped into several small pieces by a steel blade. Steel-cut oats are minimally processed, thereby preserving the natural kernel of the grain, and they have a delicious nutty flavor. Chopping the kernel into a few small pieces of oats makes this type of oat kernel perfect for cooking up a stick-to-your-ribs bowl of chewy oatmeal. Steel-cut oats are often imported from Scotland or Ireland and are available in round metal tins. My favorite is McCann's Irish oatmeal. Steel-cut oats are highly nutritious, and although they require a bit of time to cook on the stovetop, for the oat aficionado the flavor and texture of this type of oatmeal are well worth the wait.

ROLLED OATS

Rolled oats are what most Americans know as oatmeal, the kind sold in the familiar round cardboard boxes. Rolled oats consist of whole oat groats that have been steamed (a process that imparts a nutty flavor and retards rancidity), dried, sliced, and then flattened with large rollers, producing quicker-cooking flakes of oats. Note that rolled oats are still a whole grain because they retain the three key parts of the kernel: the bran layer, the germ, and the endosperm. Rolled oats can be purchased in three forms, differentiated by cooking time:

- Old-fashioned rolled oats, where either the entire grain is rolled or the grain is thickly cut and then rolled.
- Quick-cooking, where the oats have first been cut more finely and then rolled so that the flakes are smaller and thinner than old-fashioned.
- Instant, where the grains are cut thinnest of all, is actually precooked, then dehydrated and rolled. Many instant varieties come with unnecessary additives such as sugar, salt, and other flavorings. The fact that they are precooked makes them convenient but mushy and less flavorful compared to less processed oats such as steel-cut.

Of the three types of rolled oats, the old-fashioned is the most desirable. Although it takes longer to cook, it contains more beta-glucan. Incidentally, oat flour is made from either rolled oats or oat groats that have been milled to a powder.

Cheerios: One Oat Alternative

"I don't like the idea of eating bland oatmeal for breakfast every day!" a patient said, and then divulged that she truly enjoys eating her kids' Cheerios instead. In our fast-paced world, if the time commitment or the taste of the less processed oatmeal is not for you, then Cheerios are a fine alternative. In fact, a study proclaiming the cholesterol-lowering benefits of Cheerios in a group of Hispanic Americans was recently published in the *Journal of the American Dietetic Association.* One hundred and fifty-two volunteers with high LDL cholesterol levels were randomly divided into two groups. Both groups followed an NCEP Step 1 diet for six weeks. One group consumed two 1½-ounce servings of Cheerios per day (providing a daily dose of 3 grams of beta-glucan), whereas the other group instead ate two similar-sized servings of a regular corn cereal. The Cheerios group reduced their LDL cholesterol by 5.3 percent compared to no difference in the corn cereal group. The results clearly demonstrate the power of beta-glucan in lowering LDL cholesterol.

Note: One cup of Cheerios contains a mere 1 gram of beta-glucan. To obtain the 3-gram daily goal, you would need to eat two full bowls (1½ cups each) of Cheerios. That's a lot of Cheerios. If you take the Cheerios route, I recommend adding in powdered oat bran somewhere else in your day—or maybe even sprinkling it on your Cheerios—as oat bran is the most concentrated source of beta-glucan.

Source: Wahida Karmally et al., "Cholesterol-Lowering Benefits of Oat-Containing Cereal in Hispanic Americans," *Journal of the American Dietetic Association* 105 (2005): 967–970.

OAT BRAN

Oat bran is the isolated outer layer of the kernel; it is the most concentrated source of the soluble fiber, an almost pure source of beta-glucan, but a little gummy, to say the least. If you can tough it out, eat oat bran any way you can because oat bran is your best bet for getting that beta-glucan in. Experiment with concentrated oat bran. Try baking with it, adding it into muffins, breads, or pancake batter. Or simply cook it up as a hot cereal for breakfast mixed with rolled oats and soy milk. The main message here is that the more processed the oats are, the less beta-glucan the product will contain.

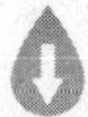 Oats: A Comparison

Type of Oat	Characteristics	Nutrition Rating	Cooking/Serving Suggestions
Groats	Oat grains that have been minimally processed (cleaned, dried, cooled, and hulls completely removed)	*****	As a breakfast cereal or in stuffing
Steel-cut	Groats that have been sliced into several pieces	*****	As a breakfast cereal
Rolled			
1. Old-fashioned	Groats cut into thick, large pieces before steaming and rolling, resulting in the thickest flakes	****	Breakfast cereal, baked goods (cookies, muffins, pancakes, and breads)
2. Quick-cooking	Oats cut into finer slices than old-fashioned oats before steaming and rolling, resulting in thinner flakes	***	Breakfast cereal, baked goods (cookies, muffins, pancakes, and breads)
3. Instant	Oats cut into the thinnest slices and then partially cooked before rolling	**	Breakfast cereal
Oat flour	Either groats or rolled oats ground into flour	****	Baked goods
Oat bran	The outer layer of the groat	****	As a breakfast cereal or added to baked goods
Some popular brands of oat products: Quaker, McCann's, Mother's, Erewhon, Nature's Path, and Bob's Red Mill.			

GOVERNMENT-RECOMMENDED

So convinced is the government of the health benefits of oats and other whole grains that in 1999 products containing them qualified for a coveted FDA health claim. Pick up any whole-grain food at your local grocery store and you will see these words: "Diets rich in whole grain foods and other plant foods low in total fat, saturated fat, and cholesterol may reduce the risk of heart disease and certain cancers."[16]

Adding to oats' claim to fame is that they were the first to attain a food-specific health claim. On January 21, 1997, the FDA granted a health claim that reads: "Soluble fiber from foods such as oat bran, rolled oats or oatmeal, and whole oat flour, as part of a diet low in saturated fat and cholesterol, may reduce the risk of heart disease." The FDA concluded, based on an extensive review of the current science, that at least 3 grams of beta-glucan per day from oats should be consumed to bring about a drop in cholesterol.

FILLING THE PRESCRIPTION

Reaching the government-recommended daily goal of beta-glucan is easy. Use the chart on page 69 to make sure your daily intake adds up to at least 3 grams.

Nothing beats the convenience of instant oatmeal, but be careful which type you buy. Quaker has a product called Take Heart Instant Oatmeal (160 calories per packet). Don't be misled by the slick marketing campaigns, as one packet of either type of instant oatmeal has only an extra 0.5 grams of soluble fiber, which may or may not be the beta-glucan variety. Better to buy the cheaper plain instant packets and then add in a couple of spoonfuls of oat bran. This way, you'll get the needed beta-glucan fiber and pay less at the checkout counter.

Tired of Oats? Eat Barley Instead

For those days when you just can't bear to eat another bowl of oatmeal, substitute barley. Barley is the only other grain that can effectively diminish LDL cholesterol levels and contains just as much soluble fiber as oats (about 25 percent of the fiber in the barley kernel is the soluble type)—and even more total dietary fiber. Whole-grain barley is highly nutritious, full of important vitamins and minerals. About 3 percent of the kernel is fat—the healthy long-chain polyunsaturated type. Within the fat is a large concentration of heart-healthy vitamin E, containing powerful antioxidant compounds called tocopherols and tocotrienols (two subgroups of the vitamin E family).

Just as with oats, the cholesterol-cutting mechanism in barley has been attributed to a high beta-glucan content, and both animal and human studies have demonstrated that beta-glucan from barley significantly lowers LDL cholesterol. Researchers evaluating the effects of barley in hamsters with high cholesterol showed a dose-dependent response—the more beta-glucan administered, the greater the reduction in LDL cholesterol. Perhaps more important, scientists discovered that barley has a powerful dampening effect on the liver's main cholesterol production enzyme, HMG-CoA reductase, the same mechanism that cholesterol-lowering statin drugs use.

The healthiest type of barley is the whole-grain variety, also called hulled barley. When shopping for barley, choose this variety over the quick-cooking or pearled versions. The darker in color the variety, the greater the amount of bran retained. On a recent trip to my local Whole Foods Market, I found gold-colored whole-grain hulled barley, the healthier kind, as well as a deeply colored "purple prairie" type of organically grown barley, another great choice. Swelling up into small dumplings and with a tongue-popping factor similar to caviar, this grain will surely add to your culinary delight. Because barley kernels contain an ample amount of heart-healthy fats that are easily oxidized, it's best to keep them stored in the refrigerator.

Source: H. Ho et al., "A Systematic Review and Meta-Analysis of Randomized Controlled Trials of the Effect of Barley β-glucan on LDL-C, Non-HDL-C and ApoB for Cardiovascular Disease Risk Reduction." *European Journal of Clinical Nutrition* 70 (2016): 1239–1245, https://doi.org/10.1038/ejcn.2016.89.

On the road and just can't seem to get that oatmeal in? See if a local café sells oatmeal on its breakfast menu or has a morning oatmeal bar.

Remember, you can also replace your daily oats with barley for lunch (a steaming bowl of mushroom barley soup, maybe) or dinner (perhaps as a delicious accompaniment to grilled fish). Don't have that extra hour-plus to spare in the morning to cook up a bowl of authentic steel-cut Irish oatmeal? Try the slow-cooker method. Pour the oats in at night, turn on the slow-cooker, and voilà—arise to a steaming hot and comforting bowl of porridge (see the recipe for Slow Cooker Oatmeal in Appendix 4).

Overnight oats are a popular way of prepping breakfast oatmeal. That's because they require zero cooking and are a grab-and-go breakfast that's delicious and nutritious. Simply place ½ cup rolled oats in a glass container and add ½ cup soy milk and 1 tablespoon chia seeds. Mix to combine. Cover with plastic wrap and refrigerate overnight. When ready to eat, add sweetener of your choice and maybe some sliced almonds and fruit. (Note that pre-packaged versions contain added sugar and artificial additives and are usually much higher in calories than homemade.)

My favorite fast, tasty, and *very* filling breakfast that provides your daily 3 grams of oat beta-glucan is two packets of Instant Quaker Oatmeal (plain) with 2 tablespoons of oat bran. Pour in a cup of soy milk, a tablespoon of dried cranberries, and your sweetener of choice, and zap in the microwave for two minutes. Sprinkle 2 tablespoons or so of ground flaxseeds on top and you've gotten in three Cholesterol Down steps before the day has barely begun!

Grain Product	Amount	Beta-glucan
McCann's Steel-cut Irish Oatmeal	½ cup dry (300 calories)	4 grams
Quaker Oat Bran	½ cup dry (150 calories)	3 grams
Old-Fashioned Quaker Oats	½ cup dry (150 calories)	2 grams
Quaker Quick-Cooking Oatmeal	½ cup dry (150 calories)	2 grams
Shiloh Farms Hulled Barley	(140 calories)	2 grams
Quaker Instant Oatmeal (plain)	1 packet (100 calories)	1 gram
Cheerios	1 cup (111 calories)	1 gram

Oats on the Internet

For more information on oats and whole grains, plus delicious oat and barley recipes, visit the following websites.

Oldways Whole Grains Council (www.wholegrainscouncil.org)
North American Millers' Association (www.namamillers.org)
US Grains Council (www.grains.org)
Quaker Oatmeal (www.quakeroatmeal.com)
McCann's Irish Oatmeal (www.mccanns.com)
FoodSubs (www.foodsubs.com/GrainOats.html)

CHAPTER 5

Step 2: Eat Almonds

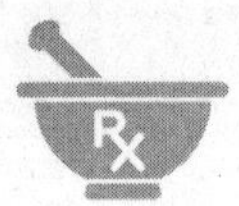

Eat a handful of almonds every day (most therapeutic dose: 1.5 ounces or approximately 30 almonds per day).

A sixty-year-old female patient of mine recently posed the following question: "My friend said if I eat almonds every day, I won't get heart disease—is this true?" Nuts, and almonds in particular, contain a plethora of healthful ingredients that have been shown to help ward off heart disease in addition to cancer—particularly colon cancer—and also to aid in weight loss. So compelling are the scientific data on heart health and almonds that the government allows food labels to carry a qualified health claim for almonds and other tree nuts.

THE NUTRITIVE POWER OF ALMONDS

It is no secret that almonds are very high in fat, but 90 percent of the fat is the heart-healthy kind—monounsaturated and polyunsaturated. One ounce of almonds contains 9 grams of monounsaturated fat, 3.5 grams of polyunsaturated fat, and an insignificant amount (1 gram) of saturated fat. These days, it's out with the old fat-phobic mentality and in with the new mantra: healthy fats are good; simple carbs are bad.

As you can see, almonds are especially high in monounsaturated fat—the same kind found in olive oil—which has been shown to lower LDL, the "bad" cholesterol. What's more, of all the tree nuts, almonds pack the most dietary fiber (more than 3 grams per ounce) and protein (6 grams per ounce), and they deliver a hefty dose of bone-building calcium (80 mg per ounce).

Almonds are unique among the nut family because they boast the highest concentration of vitamin E—in the form of alpha-tocopherol, a potent natural antioxidant. One ounce of almonds provides 50 percent of the government's recommended dietary intake. Loaded with essential minerals such as selenium, zinc, copper, calcium, iron, magnesium, and potassium plus a huge array of phytochemicals, almonds are truly nutrient-rich.

Mathew's Story

Mathew C., age twenty-three

Pre: Total cholesterol: 219 mg/dL; LDL cholesterol: 150 mg/dL

Post: Total cholesterol: 155 mg/dL; LDL cholesterol: 80 mg/dL

47 percent reduction in LDL cholesterol

Despite being a young and healthy fitness instructor, Mathew has a strong family history of high blood cholesterol and heart disease. His physician recommended a statin drug to bring his cholesterol down, but he preferred to seek a more natural treatment. Here is Mathew's story.

I thought, being young and healthy and having studied so much about the body, that I would always stay healthy. I try to eat as healthy as possible, because high cholesterol and blood pressure run in my family.

Six weeks ago, I had a blood test during a routine visit to my doctor. My doctor called a few days later and asked me to get checked out again because my cholesterol was very high (220) and my "bad" cholesterol was 150, way too high for my age and physical condition. We both thought it was a mistake because a year ago it was normal. The results came back the same. He decided he would put me on Lipitor. I have always said I would never take a medication I would have to stay on for the rest of my life, and one of my friends had recently experienced bad side effects on Lipitor, so I decided not to take it. I am into living naturally and decided that there had to be a better way to correct this problem.

My boss, a certified personal trainer, told me about a nutritionist he trains. I made an appointment and began talking to Dr. Janet that day. I started implementing her ten-part plan and followed it for an initial five-week period. It was fairly easy, and it didn't significantly alter my diet or my lifestyle. And the plan worked! My cholesterol is now down to 150 (my "bad" cholesterol is at 80), and I feel like my insides are cleaner and always fresh, based on being extremely regular.

I would suggest that anyone with high cholesterol consider giving this plan a shot. It is not difficult to follow. Along with lowering your cholesterol, it can keep you living longer just adding more natural products to your everyday diet.

THE FDA RECOMMENDS EATING ALMONDS TO PREVENT HEART DISEASE

Almonds are good for the heart, and the government wants people to know that. The FDA recommends eating almonds to prevent heart disease. Nuts—specifically almonds, hazelnuts, pecans, pistachios, walnuts, and peanuts—can now carry a label stating, "Scientific evidence suggests, but does not prove, that eating 1.5 ounces per day of most nuts, such as almonds, as part of a diet low in saturated fat and cholesterol may reduce the risk of heart disease." The qualified nature of the claim means that there are enough data out there for the FDA to state that eating a daily handful of nuts may reduce your risk for heart disease. The heart health benefits of almonds are confirmed by several top health agencies such as the American Heart Association; the National

Heart, Lung, and Blood Institute; and the most recent U.S. Dietary Guidelines, which have long touted the benefits of including nuts as a part of a heart-healthy diet.

SCIENTIFIC EVIDENCE LINKS ALMONDS TO HEART HEALTH

According to a scientific review of the effect of eating nuts on cholesterol written by a top researcher, Dr. Gary Fraser of Loma Linda University in California, four of the best large-scale studies have shown that eating nuts on a regular basis can lower your risk for heart disease by up to 50 percent.[1] Additional proof comes from the famous Seventh-Day Adventist Study, which analyzed eating habits of more than 31,000 individuals living in California. The study found that those eating nuts five or more times per week decreased their risk of dying from heart disease by 52 percent.[2]

But what about the cholesterol-cutting effects of *almonds* in particular? The buzz from a slew of research studies suggests that eating almonds can lower your LDL without a concurrent reduction in the level of "good" HDL cholesterol. Here is a synopsis of a few of the almond studies.

Adding almonds to your diet has been shown not only to reduce LDL-C levels but also to maintain HDL-C levels. A recent extensive review of the effects of eating almonds provides concrete evidence that the use of this simple nutritional strategy effectively manages known major risk factors for heart disease (such as elevated LDL and low HDL cholesterol).[3]

The effect on LDL cholesterol levels of replacing saturated fat with healthful almond fat was investigated by a group of scientists in Australia.[4] Sixteen men with normal cholesterol levels were placed on a typical Australian diet for three weeks (reference diet) and then switched over to an almond diet (where most of the saturated fat was replaced with approximately 3 ounces of raw almonds a day) for an additional period of three weeks. The results showed that adding almonds (and subtracting saturated fat) specifically targeted LDL cholesterol, as LDL dropped

10 percent—from an average of 140 mg/dL to 125 mg/dL—while the level of "good" HDL cholesterol remained unchanged. The researchers concluded that the replacement of artery-clogging saturated fat with healthful monounsaturated-fat-rich almonds not only lowers LDL but is an ideal strategy for preventing LDL from becoming oxidized, a recognized step in the atherosclerotic process.

Another research study, conducted at Loma Linda University in California, has also confirmed that eating almonds can make a dent in your LDL level.[5] Researchers placed twenty-five healthy subjects on one of three types of diets for four weeks: (1) a traditional Step 1 National Cholesterol Education Program (NCEP) diet without almonds, (2) a Step 1 diet with the addition of a daily dose of approximately 1 ounce of almonds, or (3) a Step 1 diet with approximately 2½ ounces of almonds. Compared to the traditional Step 1 diet and the Step 1 diet plus 1 ounce of almonds daily, the high-almond diet (2½ ounces) reduced LDL by 7 percent. According to the study authors, a 7 percent decrease in LDL translates into a reduction of about 11 percent in the incidence of cardiovascular disease. In fact, this particular study showed a dose-dependent response, meaning the more almonds the subjects ate, the greater their drop in LDL cholesterol.

Raw, roasted, or as almond butter, any way you eat them is going to get your "bad" cholesterol down! That's the finding from a group of researchers out of Stanford who compared the cholesterol-lowering effect of three different forms of almonds on cholesterol level.[6] Thirty-eight volunteers with high cholesterol were placed on a heart-healthy diet that included approximately 3½ ounces of almonds in one of the following three forms: roasted and salted, raw, or as almond butter. At the end of the four-week test period, it was shown that all three forms of almonds were effective at cutting LDL cholesterol, with the largest drop seen in the raw almond group (12 percent) versus a 7 percent drop in the roasted and almond butter groups.

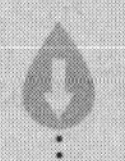

Almond Intake Lowers LDL

A recent meta-analysis of twenty-six randomized clinical trials analyzing 1,750 subjects was performed to assess the role of almond intake on LDL cholesterol levels and other heart health parameters, making it the most comprehensive and largest study on the subject ever completed. The statistical analysis clearly proves that regular almond intake significantly lowers LDL cholesterol. The researchers concluded that almonds contain a diversity of bioactive constituents that orchestrate numerous physiological and metabolic processes conducive to heart health. More specifically, almonds (with the skin) are rich in healthy fat, vitamins (with high levels of vitamin E), minerals (such as magnesium), fiber, antioxidants, and other bioactive compounds (such as arginine, phytophenols, and phytosterols), which are responsible for the heart health benefits of eating almonds.

Source: M. Morvaridzadeh et al., "The Effect of Almond Intake on Cardiometabolic Risk Factors, Inflammatory Markers, and Liver Enzymes: A Systematic Review and Meta-Analysis," *Phytotherapy Research* 36 (2022): 4325–4344.

For targeting LDL cholesterol, getting your fat from almonds as opposed to olive oil or butter appears to be the best strategy. American, Canadian, and Italian researchers collaborated on this study comparing an almond-based diet to an olive-oil-based diet and a dairy-based diet to observe effects on subjects' cholesterol level.[7] Forty-five adults with high cholesterol were all placed on a similar "background diet" with the same percentages of carbohydrate, fat, and protein. The difference in the diets was the addition of either approximately 3½ ounces of raw almonds (almond diet), approximately 1½ ounces of olive oil plus cottage cheese and crackers (olive oil diet), or approximately 3 ounces of cheddar cheese, 1 ounce of butter, and crackers (control diet). After four weeks on the respective diets, it was determined that LDL cholesterol dropped from an initial 166 mg/dL to 141 mg/dL in the almond group (15 points) versus a decline of 9 points in the olive oil diet and compared to an increase of 8 points in the control diet. Thus, this study showed that an almond-based diet is superior to an olive-oil-based diet in targeting LDL cholesterol.

IN A NUTSHELL, HOW DO ALMONDS LOWER LDL?

A daily dose of almonds is thought to battle LDL cholesterol and heart disease on several fronts.

Method of Attack #1. As noted previously, almonds contain an especially high amount of monounsaturated fat—in particular, a type known as oleic acid, an omega-9 fatty acid. Scientists think that this type of fat becomes incorporated into the core of the LDL molecule, changing the shape such that it binds more easily to LDL receptors. The greater the enrichment of LDL with unsaturated fatty acids, the greater the binding of LDL with LDL receptors on the liver.

As we've seen in prior chapters, the body's main way of lowering blood levels of LDL is by increasing LDL clearance through LDL receptors. Thus, eating nuts enhances the affinity of the LDL particle for the LDL receptor, which may be the central mechanism responsible for the consistent LDL-lowering effect observed in study after study of individuals regularly consuming almonds, walnuts, pecans, and other kinds of nuts.

Another point to consider regarding the healthy fat contained in almonds is that they contain phytosterols (discussed in depth in Chapter 10), a plant substance known to effectively cut cholesterol when consumed in high concentrations.

Method of Attack #2. Almonds contain a large amount of dietary fiber, the highest amount of dietary fiber of all the tree nuts. High-fiber diets are consistently linked with lower cholesterol levels and a reduced risk of heart disease.[8]

Method of Attack #3. Almonds contain antioxidants—including two particularly powerful types, flavonoids and vitamin E—which help prevent oxidation, a precursor to plaque buildup (atherosclerosis) and ultimately a heart attack. Studies have shown that thanks to their high antioxidant content, eating almonds significantly lowers your risk of death from heart disease.

How do we know that eating flavonoid-rich foods protects us against heart disease? Researchers at the University of Sydney in Australia performed a meta-analysis (a statistical technique analyzing a group of similar studies in an effort to draw one main conclusion) of seven large-scale studies examining flavonoid intake and risk of death from heart disease. They concluded the more flavonoids people included in their diets, the less likely they were to succumb to or die from a heart attack.[9] The researchers suggested that individuals should increase the amount of flavonoid-rich foods in their diet as a strategy for heart disease prevention.

How exactly do flavonoids work in the arteries to fight heart disease? Scientists in Israel found that antioxidants, such as plant-derived flavonoids found in high concentrations in almond skins, battle highly reactive oxygen molecules called free radicals (dangerous substances that break apart LDL particles and instigate plaque buildup) to stop atherosclerosis in its tracks.[10]

Do the flavonoids in almonds work alone to stop LDL from breaking apart? Research on hamsters out of the Antioxidants Research Laboratory at the Jean Mayer USDA Human Nutrition Research Center on Aging in Boston showed that, in fact, flavonoids partnering with vitamin E may be the secret to almonds' ability to protect LDL cholesterol and prevent death from heart disease.[11] As mentioned earlier, almonds are a uniquely rich source of vitamin E, another powerful antioxidant. Vitamin E is found in the internal fat portion of the almonds, whereas flavonoids are located mostly in the skin. After almonds are eaten, the vitamin E and flavonoids are incorporated into the LDL particle, where they thwart the deadly breakdown of LDL (the step that perpetuates inflammation in the artery wall). Thus, vitamin E and flavonoids work together to protect cells from free radical damage as well as prevent LDL from being attacked by oxygen, providing a one-two punch against atherosclerosis.

Method of Attack #4. Almonds contain an unusually high amount of the amino acid arginine, necessary for construction of nitric oxide. Nitric oxide relaxes arteries so they open up, lowering blood pressure in the process. Nitric oxide also decreases platelet adhesion, meaning it prevents blood platelets from sticking to the cells that line blood vessels, thereby lessening the ability of blood to clot and reducing the risk of heart attack. Plus, as discussed in the previous chapter, arginine affects LDL receptors, promoting an increase in LDL clearance from the bloodstream.

VITAMIN E: THE SECRET WEAPON

Vitamin E is an essential fat-soluble vitamin, which, as already mentioned, functions as an antioxidant in the human body. The fat-soluble nature of vitamin E gives it the edge over water-soluble antioxidants such as vitamin C, because it allows vitamin E to be transported through the blood *inside* the LDL molecule, where it has the best strategic position for defense against the corrosion of LDL within the arterial wall. Interestingly, scientists from the Harvard School of Public Health have found that the dangerous form of LDL—when particles become small and dense—has actually become depleted of vitamin E, which explains its predisposition to rapid oxidation and the progressive plaque-building sequence.[12]

AVOID VITAMIN E SUPPLEMENTS

"Can't I just take a vitamin E pill to get the heart benefits?" you might ask. Not according to these headlines, including "High Use of Vitamin E Linked to Heart Trouble" (*St. Petersburg Times,* August 1, 2005). How's that for a total reversal in health advice? One study, in the

January 2005 issue of *Annals of Internal Medicine,* reported that swallowing more than 400 IU of vitamin E in supplement form daily actually increases risk of death from all causes.[13] Additional research published in the prestigious British medical journal *Lancet* found that popping a daily vitamin E supplement of 600 mg did not stave off the likelihood of a heart attack in a study of more than 20,000 high-risk adults.[14] Although vitamin E is an important antioxidant, taking it in supplement form does not appear to confer protection against atherosclerosis, whereas eating foods rich in vitamin E, such as almonds, does. Why? There are possibly hundreds of additional components in the whole food that work synergistically with vitamin E to fend off disease.

These headlines on vitamin E only drive home the point of getting your E from food as opposed to supplements. Take a look at data from the Iowa Women's Health Study to back up this notion. Researchers assessed the diets of a group of more than 34,000 postmenopausal women from 1986 to 1992.[15] The researchers found that those who consumed the most vitamin E from foods (at least 10 IU of vitamin E per day) were 60 percent less likely to die of a stroke than those eating the least amount (5 IU or less per day). Consuming vitamin E supplements, however, did not appear to offer any protection against succumbing to a stroke.

More recent advice from the Office of Dietary Supplements at the National Institutes of Health (NIH) states that vitamin E naturally present in food is not harmful and does not need to be limited. In supplement form, however, high doses of vitamin E might increase the risk of bleeding (by reducing the blood's ability to form clots after a cut or injury) and of hemorrhagic stroke. The NIH has placed an upper limit for adults of 1,000 mg/day for supplements of either natural or synthetic vitamin E. Some research suggests that taking vitamin E supplements even below these upper limits might cause harm. In one study, for example, men who took 400 IU (180 mg) of synthetic vitamin E each day for several years had an increased risk of prostate cancer.[16]

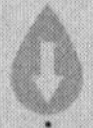

Walnuts Versus Almonds

Walnuts are a highly nutritious nut and, like almonds, have been proven to lower LDL cholesterol. Experimental research in which either almonds or walnuts were substituted for traditional fats has demonstrated significant reductions in LDL cholesterol, from 8 to 12 percent. Walnuts contain a large cache of heart-healthy omega-3 fatty acids and have a high concentration of disease-fighting antioxidants. In addition to vitamin E, walnuts contain the antioxidant resveratrol, the same ingredient that gives red wine its heart-healthy reputation. Resveratrol protects the heart by preventing the oxidation of LDL as well as attenuating the inflammatory process in the inner arterial wall.

The main difference between almonds and walnuts lies in their fatty acid profiles. Almonds contain more monounsaturated fat, mostly omega-9 fatty acids, like the fat found in olive oil. Walnuts contain more polyunsaturated fats, omega-3 fatty acids similar to those in flaxseeds. So, which is better at lowering cholesterol? One study from Australia set out to answer this question. After a nine-week period, researchers found that the almond group decreased LDL by 10 percent and the walnut group decreased LDL by 9 percent, suggesting that walnuts may be as effective in lowering LDL as almonds.

So, if you're tired of your daily dose of almonds or simply don't like them, feel free to substitute an ounce of walnuts, about fourteen halves, as a practical cardioprotective eating strategy.

Source: Mavis Abbey et al., "Partial Replacement of Saturated Fatty Acids with Almonds or Walnuts Lowers Total Plasma Cholesterol and Low-Density-Lipoprotein Cholesterol," *American Journal of Clinical Nutrition* 59 (1994): 995–999.

CAUTIONS FOR EATING NUTS

Nuts taste great, but there is one small caveat: nuts are high in calories and fat, albeit the healthy kind, so if eaten in excess they will promote weight gain. In our world of surplus calorie consumption, take note that almonds pack about 150 to 200 calories per ounce, and it is all too easy to go overboard. This prescription is not a license to overeat; you will need to compensate for the extra calories. Be prepared to cut out some other food from your day so that you don't add pounds as you subtract LDL. If you typically snack on less nutritious foods such as chips or pretzels, substituting a handful of almonds is a tasty, satisfying treat and a much more nutritious snack.

Because nuts are plant foods, they are naturally free of cholesterol. However, some varieties are extremely high in saturated fat (one of the three dietary evils you should try to avoid—the other two are cholesterol and trans fat). Brazil nuts, cashews, and macadamia nuts all contain a hefty dose of saturated fat in addition to their supply of healthy fat. Another admonition regarding nuts is that children younger than age two can easily choke on them, so parents should avoid feeding nuts to small children. Don't buy salted nuts, as the sweet flavor that surfaces during the dry-roasting process makes the addition of salt for extra taste completely unnecessary.

Nuts and Allergies: A Strong Warning

Nuts and peanuts (a legume) are two of the top eight major food allergens—fish, shellfish, eggs, wheat, milk, and soy are the others. These foods, including nuts, and especially peanuts, can trigger a severe allergic reaction in some people, which can be fatal. In fact, of all the foods people are allergic to, tree nuts and peanuts are the leading causes of death, so those allergic to nuts should obviously avoid eating them.

There has been a virtual explosion of nut allergies in children over the last few decades, and no one knows exactly why. While it is quite common for children to outgrow some types of allergies, when it comes to nuts, shellfish, and eggs the prognosis is often not as bright. This is a mounting health concern, as nut allergies are also common in adults, with over 3 million Americans having reported allergies to both tree nuts and peanuts. So, if you are allergic to nuts, pay particular attention to processed foods and scrutinize food labels, watch out for cross contamination, ask questions at restaurants, and always carry an epinephrine pen, just in case.

Sources: National Institute of Allergy and Infectious Diseases, www.niaid.nih.gov/; Scott H. Sicherer et al., "Prevalence of Peanut and Tree Nut Allergy in the United States Determined by Means of Random Digit Dial Telephone Survey: A 5-Year Follow-Up Study," *Journal of Allergy and Clinical Immunology* 112, no. 6 (December 2003): 1203–1207.

FILLING THE PRESCRIPTION

Eat a handful of almonds (1 ounce, or approximately twenty-three almonds) every day. There are two types of almonds, sweet and bitter. The bitter variety contains a poisonous substance called prussic acid and therefore its sale is forbidden in the United States. Processing bitter almonds detoxifies the prussic acid and allows for production of flavor extracts. Americans are most familiar with the sweet variety, readily available in supermarkets and natural food stores.

Almonds can be purchased in a number of different forms: blanched (skin removed) or whole (brown skin left intact), shelled or unshelled, sliced or slivered, dry-roasted or oil-roasted, salted or smoked or spiced. Your best bet is to buy shelled, natural or dry-roasted (no added oils), unsalted whole almonds. The dry-roasted form makes it easier to count out your daily dose without having the tedious chore of shelling them, plus you're not getting any added fat or salt. If you choose the pre-sliced or slivered almonds, simply weigh out 1 ounce on a kitchen scale. However, try to eat almonds that have not had their skins removed because the skin contains the bulk of the flavonoids that work hand in hand with vitamin E to prevent LDL oxidation.

The high fat content of almonds makes them susceptible to spoilage; therefore, it is best to store them in an airtight container in the refrigerator. Feel free to substitute almond butter instead of eating the whole nuts. Refer to the chart below for a list of suggested products currently available and the amount necessary to fulfill your daily almond goal.

Functional Food	Amount
Whole, shelled, dry-roasted,	1 ounce, or about 23 nuts
(no added salt), natural almonds	(169 calories)
Almond butter	2 tablespoons (200 calories)
English walnuts	1 ounce, or about 14 halves (185 calories)

Almonds on the Internet

For more information on almonds or for some great recipe ideas, log on to the following websites.

Almond Board of California (www.almonds.com)
Agricultural Marketing Resource Center (www.agmrc.org/commodities-products/nuts/almonds)
International Nut & Dried Fruit Council (http://inc.nutfruit.org)
International Tree Nut Council (www.treenuts.org)

CHAPTER 6

Step 3: Eat Flaxseeds

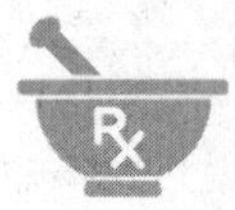

Eat 2 tablespoons of ground flaxseeds every day (3 grams of ALA).

A fifty-two-year-old female patient once said to me, "I've been eating flaxseeds since I read in Dr. Bob Arnot's book that flaxseeds help prevent breast cancer. Can they prevent heart disease, too?" The answer is yes—they are very effective at lowering your "bad" LDL cholesterol. Multiple studies in animals and a handful of clinical studies in humans have shown great promise for the use of ground flaxseeds in lowering LDL cholesterol. As an added benefit, eating flaxseeds helps protect against cancer—most notably breast, colon, and prostate (and has also been linked to increased brain function). Flaxseeds (aka linseeds) are packed with a host of nutrients including protein, iron, phosphorus, calcium, B vitamins, and vitamin E. The protein content of flaxseeds is similar to the healthy amino acid profile found in soybeans and almonds.

Flaxseeds contain high amounts of several biologically active components, earning them the coveted title of a true "superfood." A recent review[1] touts the miraculous medicinal effects of eating flaxseed on human health. According to the authors, regular consumption of flaxseed can improve cholesterol and lower blood pressure, fasting blood sugar, and insulin resistance. Moreover, flaxseed has anticancer and antioxidant properties. It can significantly reduce the intensity of symptoms associated with menopause, constipation, and mental fatigue; improve skin condition; and accelerate wound healing.

Alma's Story

Dr. Alma B., age eighty-two

Pre: Total cholesterol: 212 mg/dL; LDL cholesterol: 144 mg/dL

Post: Total cholesterol: 169 mg/dL; LDL cholesterol: 92 mg/dL

36 percent reduction in LDL cholesterol

Alma has been taking statin drugs for over two decades. Despite this, she was unable to get her "bad" cholesterol down to her goal. Her doctor recommended she increase the dosage of her statin drug, but she refused, as she has had trouble with leg cramps, a side effect from the medication, in the past. Here's what she has to say.

I am a psychoanalyst and an author. I have had very high cholesterol since I was first tested at the age of fifty. At its highest, it reached over 350. My physician told me that my life was in danger.

I have been taking cholesterol-lowering drugs for years. While my cholesterol levels dropped, they caused intense cramping in my legs and more recently in my hands. Despite careful monitoring of my diet and a daily dosage of Lipitor (10 to 20 mg), my cholesterol levels remained abnormally high, until recently, when I began to follow Dr. Janet Brill's plan for lowering cholesterol, together with taking 10 mg of Lipitor daily. Her suggestions worked brilliantly. At my most recent reading, I found my cholesterol level had dropped to 169, LDL 92, the first time in my life that I was ever able to get my "bad" LDL cholesterol under 130. I am happy that now I will not have to take the higher dosage of Lipitor with its side effect of cramps. I am thrilled with the wonderful results of Dr. Brill's program.

THE BENEFITS OF OMEGA-3 FATTY ACIDS

When it comes to the health-promoting properties of flaxseeds, most experts agree that it is the rich omega-3 fatty acid content and the high concentration of lignan and soluble fiber that confer the benefits. Let's look first at the special fat in flax.

WHAT ARE ESSENTIAL FATTY ACIDS, AND WHERE DO THEY COME FROM?

A full 35 percent of a flaxseed's weight comes from oil. The oil has a unique composition: it is a virtual storage vat of polyunsaturated essential fatty acids. The body does not manufacture essential fatty acids, so we must consume them in our diets. A deficiency can result in skin changes (flaking, itching, and the development of sores), hair loss, intestinal problems, and growth retardation in children.

Nutritionists often refer to essential fatty acids as protective fats, of which there are two main groups, both essential for life: omega-3 and omega-6 fatty acids. Each type of essential fatty acid has what is considered a parent acid, alpha-linolenic acid (ALA) for omega-3 and linoleic acid (LA) for omega-6. For the purposes of this book, you need to know that the *omega-3 fatty acids confer extremely powerful heart-protective effects.* Read on to learn why eating omega-3 fat is vital for heart health.

Although essential fatty acids can come from meat and fish, plants are their main source—including water plants such as phytoplankton and algae. LA (omega-6) is found mainly in seeds, nuts, and legumes. Most Americans get an oversupply of omega-6s from the omega-6-rich vegetable oils such as safflower oil, soybean oil, and cottonseed oil that pervade our food supply. At the same time, we get an undersupply of healthful omega-3 fats, which are not nearly as plentiful in our food supply as omega-6 fats. This fatty acid imbalance is a troublesome situation, as it leads to negative health ramifications. One must therefore make a concerted effort to boost omega-3 fatty acid intake, which is not an easy task given that only a select few sources provide the special omega-3 fat ALA. These sources include English walnuts, some wild leafy greens, soy, canola oil, and flaxseed—the richest plant source of the omega-3 fatty acid ALA.

TWO TYPES OF OMEGA-3 FATTY ACIDS

There are two varieties of omega-3 fatty acids: the short-chain form, such as ALA, found in plants, and the long-chain forms, found in fish, seafood, and plants from the sea (microalgae and seaweed). The only type of omega-3 fatty acid found in flaxseed is the short-chain form, ALA. This form differs from the more physiologically active long-chain types of omega-3 fats (eicosapentaenoic acid, or EPA, and docasahexaenoic acid, or DHA) found mainly in fatty fish.

It is well known that atherosclerosis is an inflammatory disorder; therefore, there has been much recent research interest involving the anti-inflammatory effects of omega-3 fatty acids. Most of this research linking omega-3 fat consumption with heart health has been done with the kind of fat found in fish oil, not flaxseeds. However, the two types of omega-3 fatty acids are similar enough to infer that those from flaxseeds work in much the same way to fight inflammation, and new research supports this conclusion.

For example, Harvard researchers examined data from a subset of 727 women participating in the famed Nurses' Health Study—one of the largest prospective studies to investigate risk factors for chronic disease in women.[2] The scientists wanted to know if there was any relationship between the nurses' dietary omega-3 fatty acid intake (from fish or plant sources) and blood levels of various markers for inflammation. It was determined that not only did eating a diet high in omega-3 fats decrease inflammation but that indeed there was a significant inverse relationship between ALA (the short-chain fatty acid found in flaxseeds) and the level of blood inflammatory markers.

Data continue to accumulate showing that ALA (the short-chain omega-3 fatty acid), derived specifically from flaxseeds, exhibits substantial cardioprotective effects. Researchers at Pennsylvania State University looked at how ALA works to prevent heart disease.[3] The scientists placed subjects with high cholesterol on a diet rich in ALA derived primarily from flaxseed oil and walnuts. Following the test period, blood was drawn and analyzed for levels of arterial inflammation. The results? Subjects exhibited significantly reduced inflammatory markers such as C-reactive protein (you want this as low as possible) and fewer adhesion molecules lining the arteries, meaning less plaque formation.

In animals, the effect of omega-3 fatty acids versus omega-6 fatty acids on blood vessel health was investigated in a study of mice bred to rapidly develop atherosclerosis and blood clots. Japanese researchers demonstrated that the mouse diet highest in ALA (omega-3), derived from flaxseed oil, was the most effective in suppressing atherosclerosis and the formation of blood clots.[4] Conversely, the mouse diet highest in LA (omega-6), derived from safflower oil, showed the greatest degree of plaque formation and a much more pronounced tendency for the blood to clot.

DIET MAKES A BIG DIFFERENCE WHEN IT COMES TO ESSENTIAL FATTY ACIDS

The body uses essential fatty acids to produce hormone-like substances called eicosanoids. These chemicals regulate blood pressure and the immune system as well as modulate allergic and inflammatory responses. Some types of eicosanoids are highly inflammatory, linked to numerous health disorders including cardiovascular disease, whereas others are anti-inflammatory and immune-boosting in nature. Humans can manipulate the type of eicosanoids formed simply by changing what we eat.

In the body, we convert the parent essential fatty acids of the omega-3 (ALA) and omega-6 (LA) families into longer-chain and more physiologically active forms. (The conversion of ALA into longer-chain fatty acids is very limited, however.) Eicosanoids can be formed only from these more developed long-chain fatty acids. Therefore, the parent omega-3s and omega-6s fight for the enzymes required to make the conversions to these long-chain fatty acid eicosanoid precursors. This is referred to as functioning through competitive pathways, meaning that whichever essential fatty acid—omega-3 or omega-6—has the highest concentration wins the enzymes to make the conversion. So, the balance in the type of eicosanoids produced shifts depending on the type of food you eat. If you eat more omega-3s by eating flaxseeds, for example, your body will produce the more healthful anti-inflammatory eicosanoids. Eating more omega-6s, found in, say, safflower oil, will result in greater production of the inflammatory disease-promoting eicosanoids. This simple dietary maneuver—increasing omega-3 intake and decreasing omega-6—can greatly affect your health and well-being.

Tips for Consuming More Omega-3s and Fewer Omega-6s

1. Eat your daily dose of ground flaxseeds (2 tablespoons), which will provide about 3 grams of omega-3 ALA, an amount that exceeds the 2.2 grams a day recommended by the National Institutes of Health.
2. Flaxseed oil is one of the few known plant sources of omega-3 fatty acids, so try using some in place of other oils. Flaxseed oil is great in salad dressings or as a flavoring for vegetables or grains.
3. Add a tablespoon of canola oil, another leading plant source of ALA omega-3 fatty acids, to your daily diet to get an additional 1.3 grams.
4. Eat some fish today. In terms of fish omega-3s, the National Institutes of Health has recommended a goal of 0.65 grams a day, or about 4.5 grams per week, of long-chain omega-3s. Oily fish, such as salmon, mackerel, sardines, herring, and rainbow trout, provide a hefty dose of these marine omega-3 fatty acids (between 1.2 and 2.5 grams per 3½-ounce serving).

5. **Limit your intake of vegetable oils rich in omega-6s: corn oil, cottonseed oil, safflower oil, sunflower oil, and soybean oil. Check your salad dressing labels because commercial dressings are frequently made with omega-6 vegetable oil.**

Source: "Workshop on the Essentiality of and Recommended Dietary Intakes for Omega-6 and Omega-3 Fatty Acids," http://ods.od.nih.gov/news/conferences/w6w3_abstracts.html.

HOW CAN YOU OBTAIN A HEALTHY BALANCE OF ESSENTIAL FATTY ACIDS?

At a National Institutes of Health (NIH) workshop, numerous nutrition experts reached a consensus that Americans should reduce dietary intake of omega-6s and increase omega-3 fat intake. Increasing omega-3 intake ensures not only cardiovascular health but optimal brain development in infants, as well as preventing inflammatory events and disease linked to excessive omega-6 fat consumption.

Nutrition and health professionals are very concerned about the typical American dietary intake ratio of omega-6 to omega-3 fatty acids of between 20:1 and 30:1. This unbalanced ratio is because omega-6 fats are ubiquitous among the processed foods so commonly consumed in the American diet. Although no specific ratio has been established by the U.S. government, many other countries and the World Health Organization (WHO) have declared health-promoting omega-6-to-omega-3 ratio goals of between 5:1 and 10:1. Japan recently changed its guidelines from a 4:1 ratio to a 2:1 ratio, and Canada recommends a ratio of between 4:1 and 10:1.[5]

LIGNAN, THE OTHER MEDICINAL COMPONENT IN FLAX

Flaxseeds are unique among plants not only for their rich omega-3 fatty acid content but also because they contain the highest concentration of lignan, another key ingredient related to heart health. Flaxseeds contain up to 800 times the amount of lignan found in other oil seeds. Lignans are a type of phytoestrogen, meaning they are hormone-like plant substances with weak estrogen-like effects, and are chemically similar to the isoflavones found in soy.

Lignans are metabolized in the human intestine by friendly bacterial flora into two hormone-like compounds, called enterodiol and enterolactone, and are absorbed and circulated in the bloodstream. Here they exert powerful antioxidant effects that inhibit the process of atherosclerosis, cut LDL cholesterol, prevent certain types of cancers (specifically the hormone-related breast and prostate cancers), and can contribute to increased brain function much like estrogen replacement therapy.

FLAXSEEDS LOWER LDL

The scientific data are out there: flaxseed consumption lowers blood LDL cholesterol levels in individuals with either high or normal blood cholesterol levels. The majority of published clinical trials with humans show that eating a daily dose of flaxseeds, between 2 and 6 tablespoons, can lower LDL cholesterol up to 18 percent.[6] *Note that for LDL cholesterol lowering, it is consumption of the whole flaxseed and not flaxseed oil that confers this positive effect.* One study out of the University of Illinois at Chicago involved almost forty postmenopausal women randomly assigned to one of two dietary regimens: a normal diet with about 4½ tablespoons (38 grams) of ground flaxseed a day in the form of a muffin or bread or a normal diet with the same amount of sunflower seeds.[7] After the six-week treatment phase, the flaxseed group demonstrated a remarkable reduction in LDL cholesterol of 15 percent, yet LDL was unchanged under the sunflower seed treatment.

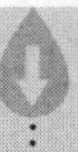

Flax exhibits strong antioxidant, anti-inflammatory, anti-clotting, blood-sugar-lowering, and blood-pressure-lowering activities, factors that contribute to its heart-healthy reputation.

HOW DO FLAXSEEDS LOWER LDL?

Flaxseeds fight heart disease and promote a noteworthy drop in LDL cholesterol in multiple ways. The bulk of the scientific research has focused on two constituents in flaxseed known to specifically target LDL metabolism: lignan and soluble fiber. Canadian researchers found that even after removing most of the fat (ALA) from the flaxseed before administering it to twenty subjects with high cholesterol, the group significantly lowered their LDL cholesterol (7 percent) without a concomitant drop in good HDL cholesterol, after three weeks.[8] As a result of the study's findings, the scientists hypothesized that while the essential fatty acids from omega-3 contribute, the primary mechanism by which flaxseed lowers LDL cholesterol is most likely the lignan component of flax or the soluble fiber—or a combination of the two. So let's begin this discussion with the top two components thought to be responsible for the strong LDL-lowering effect of eating flaxseeds: lignans and soluble fiber.

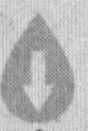

Whole Flaxseeds Affect LDL; Flaxseed Oil Does Not

Scientists recently took a close look at 26 different studies involving nearly 1,600 people to see if flaxseed really helps lower cholesterol. What they found was pretty interesting: People who ate whole flaxseeds saw their LDL cholesterol drop by an average of 7 mg/dL, while those who took flaxseed oil didn't see any improvement at all.

So, why do whole flaxseeds work better than the oil? The researchers found several reasons: Whole flaxseeds are an essential source of high-quality protein and soluble fiber, which are not found in the oil. Flaxseeds are the best source of α-linolenic acid (ALA) and are loaded with lignans (which play a role in preventing atherosclerosis and have anti-inflammatory and antioxidant properties). They also contain both soluble and insoluble dietary fibers. The fiber reduces blood glucose and cholesterol levels by delaying and reducing their absorption from the intestine.

Flax oil differs from the whole seed, as it does not contain lignan, but it can still be used to boost daily intake of omega-3 fatty acids. Because the precise cholesterol-lowering mechanism of flax has not yet been fully identified and because studies suggest the components most likely responsible for lowering cholesterol are either the lignans, the soluble fiber, or a combination of the two, you should consume the whole seed and not just the oil for maximum cholesterol-lowering benefits.

Source: C. Yang et al., "Comparisons of the Effects of Different Flaxseed Products Consumption on Lipid Profiles, Inflammatory Cytokines and Anthropometric Indices in Patients with Dyslipidemia Related Diseases: Systematic Review and a Dose–Response Meta-Analysis of Randomized Controlled Trials," *Nutrition and Metabolism* 18, no. 19 (October 2021): 91. doi:10.1186/s12986-021-00619-3.

Method of Attack #1. Fascinating research performed by Kailash Prasad on rabbits suggests that a particular lignan found in flax (scientifically known as secoisolariciresinol diglucoside, or SDG) is the major active ingredient responsible for the LDL-cutting action of flaxseed.[9] In this study, the lignan portion of flaxseeds was isolated, and rabbits were fed a cholesterol-raising rabbit chow either with or without added lignan. At the end of the eight-week test period, the lignan-fed rabbits exhibited a 35 percent reduction in LDL cholesterol compared to the control. What's more, the rabbits' aortas were examined for evidence of plaque formation. As expected, the rabbits on the high cholesterol diet had significant plaque buildup, whereas the addition of lignans reduced atherosclerotic plaque by 73 percent! According to this scientist, the powerful antioxidant activity of SDG was largely responsible for the dramatic reduction in aortic plaque observed. Thus, this lignan has demonstrated significant antioxidant properties (thwarting the oxidation of LDL cholesterol) in addition to preventing blood platelets from sticking together and clotting—both key to preventing atherosclerosis.

Another group of scientists postulated that lignans lower LDL cholesterol by impeding the actions of two key cholesterol enzymes, one involved in the production of bile acids from cholesterol (7 alpha-hydroxylase) and the other a leading player in plaque buildup (acyl CoA cholesterol transferase).[10]

Method of Attack #2. Twenty-five percent of the fiber in flaxseeds is soluble. Several ways in which most soluble fibers are believed to contribute to LDL cholesterol reduction are by increasing the excretion of bile acids, blocking cholesterol absorption, and speeding up intestinal transit time of feces. Scientists working with guinea pigs at the University of Arizona set out to determine exactly how dietary soluble fiber works to lower LDL cholesterol.[11] Soluble fiber affects the composition of VLDL secreted from the liver such that the particles have a higher content of phospholipids (and a correspondingly lower amount of cholesterol). This change in VLDL composition slows the conversion rate of VLDL to LDL, and less conversion means less circulating LDL cholesterol. Furthermore, changes in the ratio of cholesterol to phospholipids in liver cell walls as a result of soluble fiber in the diet leads to greater liver cell membrane fluidity and greater rates of cholesterol excretion from the body.

Method of Attack #3. Just as soluble fiber increases membrane fluidity, the ALA omega-3 fatty acids in flaxseeds are polyunsaturated fatty acids, and eating them has beneficial effects on cell membranes as well. Polyunsaturated fatty acids are flexible, far more pliable than stiff saturated fatty acids. An increase in the amount of polyunsaturated fats consumed keeps all cell membranes supple, including cell membranes of LDL molecules floating in the blood by increasing the flexibility of the phospholipids that comprise the bulk of the LDL outer wall. The scientific data reveal a strong connection between membrane fluidity and LDL clearance: the more fluid the membrane—meaning the greater the polyunsaturated fatty acid content—the greater the ability to clear LDL cholesterol from the bloodstream, internalize it, and degrade it.[12] Conversely, the more rigid the membrane—that is, the greater the saturated fatty acid content within the phospholipids—the less LDL cleared from the bloodstream.

Your food choices determine which type of fatty acids reside within your cells. Therefore, you should eat more omega-3 fatty acids, such as those found in flaxseeds, as they increase cell membrane fluidity, which in turn promotes cholesterol excretion.

FLAX CAUTION

Some people may be hypersensitive to flaxseed and could potentially have an allergic reaction. Obviously, if you know you are allergic to flaxseed, avoid consuming it. Flax also has a marked laxative effect (ground seeds absorb a lot of water) and, like all dietary fiber, should be added to the diet in stages to prevent gastrointestinal distress.

A high-fiber intake should be accompanied by sufficient fluid intake to prevent bowel obstruction, a highly unlikely situation. An 8-ounce glass of water taken with your daily 2 tablespoons of ground flaxseeds should be sufficient to avoid this scenario.

FILLING THE PRESCRIPTION

You can buy flaxseeds whole or pre-ground. As flaxseeds have an impenetrable outer coating, they're easier to digest in the ground-up form. Buy them whole, store them in an airtight container, and grind them on an as-needed basis just before sprinkling on your food (I use a coffee grinder). Once ground, flaxseeds go rancid quickly—their high fat content makes them susceptible to spoilage, so if you do choose the pre-ground variety, always keep them in an airtight container in the refrigerator.

You can purchase whole seeds in bulk form at your local health food store or pre-ground flaxseeds available as a dietary supplement (usually found in the vitamin section of your local supermarket). One example is Bob's Red Mill Ground Organic Flaxseed Meal. You can also order sealed ground organic flaxseed online.

There are two types of flaxseeds available for purchase: the more familiar dark brown glossy seeds and a golden-colored variety. Both are similar in terms of nutritional makeup; however, you will most likely find only the dark brown seeds readily available in supermarkets and health food stores.

Functional Food	Amount	Soluble Fiber
Whole flaxseeds (ground)	2 level tablespoons (78 calories)	2 grams

Flax on the Internet

For more information about flaxseeds, purchasing information, and some great recipes, I suggest visiting the following websites.

Flax Council of Canada (www.flaxcouncil.ca)

Prairie Flax Products, Inc. (www.prairiepremiumproducts.com)

Golden Valley Flax (www.goldenvalleyflax.com)

CHAPTER 7

Step 4: Take a Psyllium Fiber Supplement

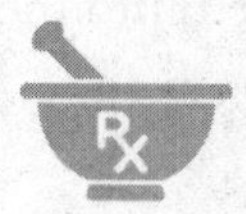

Consume 3 grams (starting dose) to 10 grams (most therapeutic dose) of psyllium husk every day.

"I don't need to take a fiber supplement. Didn't they use to market it as a laxative? I'm fine in that department . . . I'd be in the bathroom all day!" is invariably the response I get when I suggest to my patients that they take a psyllium fiber supplement on a regular basis. My response? "Don't worry, they don't increase bathroom frequency very much. But it is an easy way to keep your digestive system healthy and help you to take in dietary fiber, and believe me, it works like a charm to get your 'bad' cholesterol down!"

Could it be true—a fiber supplement that cuts cholesterol? What many people don't realize is that the active ingredient in these supplements, psyllium husk, is the most powerful LDL-lowering fiber in existence. Plus, a high-fiber diet in general has been proven to reduce risk for heart disease. A huge study[1] of close to 15,000 people strengthens the evidence that eating a high-fiber diet reduces the risk of heart disease. Higher dietary fiber intake was associated with a lower long-term cardiovascular disease risk, especially in the 20–39 and 40–59 age groups, where the reduction was most significant. More data, derived from a University of Minnesota study that pooled the results of several studies—examining data from over 300,000 men and women from the

United States and Europe—investigated the link between fiber from different foods (grains, fruits, and vegetables) and heart disease.[2] For every 10 grams of total dietary fiber intake per day, risk of heart attack dropped by an estimated 14 percent and risk of dying from the disease by 27 percent. The reduced risk was mostly attributable to soluble fiber—the same type found in psyllium husk.

In addition to lowering cholesterol, a psyllium fiber supplement promotes more regular and rapid digestion—a sign of overall health. The faster the contents of the bowel move through the gut, the fewer carcinogens, pollutants, and other toxins that will be absorbed into the cells lining the intestinal wall. In addition, a high-fiber diet helps manage diabetes and control weight.

Harry's Story

Harry B., age seventy-five

Pre: Total cholesterol: 209 mg/dL; LDL cholesterol: 123 mg/dL

Post: Total cholesterol: 157 mg/dL; LDL cholesterol: 67 mg/dL

46 percent reduction in LDL cholesterol

Harry is a survivor. First he survived the Holocaust and emigrated to Israel on the famous *Exodus* ship at the age of seventeen. Then he survived heart disease—he had a major heart attack at the age of forty-seven and open-heart surgery three months later. After his heart attack, Harry went on the Pritikin program in an effort to protect himself against the development of any additional heart problems. In the last few years, however, he strayed from the strict program, gaining back some weight, and his LDL cholesterol rose with his weight gain. His doctor had prescribed Vytorin, a newer drug that is a combination of a statin and a cholesterol absorption blocker, in an effort to get Harry's LDL down to the ultra-low LDL goal for high-risk patients. Here is what Harry had to say.

My doctor put me on this drug called Vytorin. I followed my doctor's orders and began taking Vytorin, one pill before bedtime. I live in Florida during the winter months, where I like to take long walks every day; sometimes I walk for up to two hours. After about a month and a half on the medication, I began to suffer terribly painful muscle cramps, mostly in my right calf, but only during my walks. I was in a lot of pain—so much pain that I had to stop the walking. I immediately called my doctor, and he told me to stop taking the drug.

Some time later, my daughter-in-law told me that she could lower my "bad" cholesterol without drugs or any painful side effects. I agreed to follow her diet as best I could. The only side effect I found was that I had to run to the toilet more often! I also experimented with making oatmeal cookies and added in the bran [Metamucil] plus the flaxseeds and found that the cookies were an easier way for me to get those steps in. After about a month, she asked me to go take my blood again. When she saw my results, both she and I were very happy, and I plan on continuing to follow her plan on keeping my "bad" cholesterol down. Plus, I can now enjoy my walks in Florida without any pain!

GETTING YOUR FILL OF FIBER

Unfortunately, Americans are woefully deficient in fiber intake, falling quite short of the American Heart Association's recommended 25 to 30 grams per day. The average American eats just about half that, or approximately 15 grams per day.

Why the fiber shortage on our nation's plates? Foods high in dietary fiber include whole grains, legumes, fruits, and vegetables. Few Americans eat the recommended servings of whole grains per day, and even fewer consume the amounts recommended in the 2020–2025 Dietary Guidelines for Americans: 1½- to 2-cup-equivalents of fruits and 2- to 3-cup-equivalents of vegetables per day. Keep in mind that it's not just the fiber in these foods that confers significant health benefits. Foods high in fiber also frequently contain a host of other substances such as antioxidants and phytochemicals that offer protection against disease.

WHAT ARE THE DIFFERENT TYPES OF FIBER?

In recent years, new concepts on dietary fiber have evolved. Previously, fiber was most often categorized in terms of water solubility and was divided into two main classes, soluble and insoluble. Plant foods typically contain both types, though most usually contain a greater concentration of one over the other.

- **Soluble fibers** differ chemically from insoluble fibers in that they dissolve in water. You should know, however, that not all types of soluble fiber are effective at lowering LDL cholesterol. Only those soluble fibers that carry the important characteristic of *viscosity* (the ability to form a water-holding network or bolus within the intestine that is resistant to flow) are capable of effectively reducing cholesterol. Soluble fiber is what makes oatmeal gummy, what allows pectin to gel, and what gives beans their mushy center. Soluble fiber is abundant in oats and barley (beta-glucan), purified fiber supplements made from psyllium husk (soluble fiber in the form of a gel-forming mucilage), apples (pectin), flaxseeds (also a mucilage), and beans (soluble fiber primarily in the form of gums). The high water-holding capacity of this type of fiber causes it to swell like a sponge within the intestine, pulling in water and nutrients as it travels slowly down the intestinal tract—including cholesterol and bile acids.
- **Insoluble fiber** (often termed "roughage") absorbs water, creating a bulky stool that speeds up the intestine's ability to transit the contents from end to end. Insoluble fiber differs from soluble fiber in that it does not form a gel. Good sources of insoluble fiber include wheat bran, popcorn, brown rice, and nuts. Be sure to eat the skin on potatoes and fruit with its peel to boost your insoluble fiber intake.

SOLUBLE FIBER LOWERS LDL

Most people know that eating fiber promotes regular bowel movements. But you probably didn't know that eating soluble fiber is highly effective in targeting LDL cholesterol for excretion. In fact, the FDA has allowed two soluble fiber health claims, one for oats and the other for psyllium. The FDA estimates that for every gram of soluble fiber consumed per day, total cholesterol drops between 0.5 and 2.0 percent.[3]

HOW MUCH SOLUBLE FIBER IS BEST?

For maximum LDL cholesterol lowering, the National Cholesterol Education Program advises Americans to aim for 10 to 25 grams per day of soluble fiber—not to be confused with higher total dietary fiber recommendations. Americans fall far short of this intake, with average consumption estimated at a mere 3 to 4 grams per day, so I recommend that you start with a more practical daily goal of 12 grams of soluble fiber daily, and I suggest you take psyllium husk as a supplement to aid you in attaining that goal.

Is 12 grams enough to lower LDL? Scientists of the famed Portfolio diet calculate that consuming 5 to 10 grams daily of soluble fiber lowers LDL by approximately 5 percent.[4] A review of fiber as medical nutrition therapy for high cholesterol concludes that the dose of soluble fiber needed to lower blood cholesterol levels is 12 to 30 grams per day, resulting in a 10 to 20 percent drop in total and LDL cholesterol.[5] So yes, 12 grams can make a significant difference.

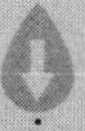

Scientists have estimated that for each gram of soluble fiber consumed from psyllium, oats, or pectin, LDL cholesterol will decrease by approximately 1.6 mg/dL. That means that you could lower your LDL from, say, 160 mg/dL to approximately 140 mg/dL, just by eating 12 grams of soluble fiber a day.

Source: Lisa Brown et al., "Cholesterol-Lowering Effects of Dietary Fiber: A Meta-Analysis," *American Journal of Clinical Nutrition* 69 (1999): 30–42.

Some of my patients say that even attaining the 12-grams-a-day goal is difficult without adding in a non-food fiber supplement—hence my decision to include supplements, such as Metamucil, in the ten-step plan. The following chart gives you an idea of how several of the Cholesterol Down steps contribute to the LDL-lowering soluble fiber prescription.

Sources of Viscous Soluble Fiber

Food or Supplement	Amount	Soluble Fiber
Metamucil (psyllium husk)	12 capsules	5.0 grams
Oatmeal	1 cup cooked (steel-cut)	3.0 grams
Okra	1 cup cooked	3.0 grams
Peas	1 cup cooked	2.6 grams
Brussels sprouts	½ cup cooked	2.6 grams
Kidney beans, pinto beans	½ cup cooked	2.4 grams
Flaxseeds	2 tablespoons (ground)	2.2 grams
Prunes	6 medium	2.0 grams
Eggplant	1 cup cooked	1.0 grams
Apple (with skin)	1 medium	0.5 grams
Almonds	1 ounce (23 almonds)	0.5 grams

Source: James W. Anderson, *Plant Fiber in Foods* (Lexington, Ky.: HCF Nutrition Research Foundation, 1990).

FERMENTABILITY, ANOTHER VIRTUE OF SOLUBLE FIBER

In addition to viscosity (the ability to form a thick liquid-like mass that is resistant to flow), many types of soluble fiber—for example, beta-glucan and psyllium—also demonstrate a characteristic called fermentability. Fermentability describes the tendency for fiber to be digested by friendly bacteria inhabiting the lower intestine.

When bacteria in the colon eat fermentable fiber, they release a by-product that gives rise to three short-chain fatty acids: propionate, butyrate, and acetate. Cells of the colon feast on butyrate in particular, a short-chain fatty acid that improves the health of these cells. Propionate and acetate are absorbed into the bloodstream. Once absorbed into the body, propionate travels to the liver, where it interferes with the production of internal cellular cholesterol. These compounds signal your liver to slow down its production of bile, a substance your body uses to digest fats. When your liver makes less bile, it forces your body to use up more of its stored cholesterol, which helps lower your overall cholesterol levels.

Propionate also lessens the ability of blood to clot, contributing further to this short-chain fatty acid's heart-healthy reputation. Bottom line: choose foods that are rich in fermentable fiber to support greater propionate production, as higher amounts are most desirable for heart health.

PSYLLIUM: BEST LDL-LOWERING SOLUBLE FIBER

Psyllium (known scientifically as a hydrophilic mucilloid) is a soluble fiber that comes from the husks of seeds of the psyllium plant *(Plantago ovata)* and also happens to be the active ingredient in some fiber supplements, such as Metamucil. (Psyllium seed husk is also known as Plantago husk.) According to scientists at the University of Wisconsin, taking psyllium (15 grams per day in the form of Metamucil) has the following healthful effects on the contents of the bowel, without greatly affecting defecation frequency: increased stool weight, faster transit time, and greater moisture content.[6] In contrast to other types of soluble fiber, several components in psyllium fiber survive transit through the colon without being fermented by bacteria. Thus, psyllium is a unique type of soluble fiber, containing enough fermentable fiber to produce large amounts of LDL-lowering propionate in addition to some unfermentable fiber that promotes healthful changes in bowel function.

FDA confirms Psyllium Is Safe and Effective for Cholesterol Reduction

Worried that taking psyllium is dangerous? Have no fear, two fibers, psyllium and β-glucan (oatmeal), have the coveted Food and Drug Administration–approved health claim for reducing the risk of cardiovascular disease. Both types of fiber lower serum cholesterol. According to the FDA, "Daily dietary intake levels of soluble fiber sources listed in this section have been associated with reduced risk coronary heart disease: (1) 3 grams or more per day of [beta]-glucan soluble fiber from either whole oats or barley, or a combination of whole oats and barley. (2) 7 grams or more per day of soluble fiber from psyllium seed husk."

Source: Code of Federal Regulations. Title 21, sec. 101.81, 2016, accessed October 2, 2025, www.ecfr.gov/current/title-21/chapter-I/subchapter-B/part-101/subpart-E/section-101.81.

THE SCIENCE OF PSYLLIUM AND CHOLESTEROL

Clinical trials using psyllium doses of 7 to 10 grams per day have consistently reported dramatic declines in LDL cholesterol, from 10 to 24 percent.[7] In a double-blind, placebo-controlled study[8] of twenty-six men, eight weeks of 3.4 grams of psyllium or cellulose placebo at mealtimes (three doses per day totaling a daily dose of approximately 10 g/day) showed remarkable results. LDL cholesterol plummeted in the psyllium group by 20.2 percent relative to baseline values. What's more, the subjects were able to stick with the psyllium treatment, and no adverse side effects were observed.

Scientists from the Metabolic Research Group at the University of Kentucky recruited forty-four men and women with high cholesterol to participate in their study investigating the effects of adding in either psyllium-enriched cereal or wheat bran flake cereal to a heart-healthy diet on cholesterol.[9] After six weeks, the subjects eating the psyllium-enriched cereal (containing approximately 3 grams of psyllium) showed a remarkable 13 percent drop in LDL cholesterol, compared to just 3 percent in the wheat bran cereal eaters. The psyllium was well tolerated by study participants, with no reported adverse side effects.

Adding more fuel to the fire, a meta-analysis of twelve studies that investigated the potential effect of psyllium-enriched cereal in subjects with high cholesterol found that those treated with the psyllium-enriched cereal exhibited significantly reduced LDL cholesterol levels, accompanied by no change in "good" HDL cholesterol, compared to control groups.[10] The findings suggest that *of all the soluble fibers, psyllium is one of the most effective for lowering LDL, with relatively few adverse side effects.*

HOW DOES PSYLLIUM WORK TO LOWER LDL CHOLESTEROL?

The impressive LDL-lowering action of psyllium is the result of several different methods of attack.

Method of Attack #1. Much like the soluble fiber in oatmeal, psyllium fiber gets rid of bile acids by physically trapping them in a large mass within the intestine, which is then excreted. When bile acids are carried out of the body as waste instead of being recycled, the liver pulls in more LDL cholesterol from the bloodstream to compensate.

Psyllium Reduces Cardiovascular Event Risk

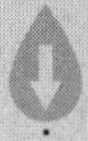

A new and exciting finding from researchers in China confirms the dramatic heart health benefits of consuming psyllium seed husk. The recent meta-analysis of twenty-nine randomized clinical trials included 2,769 participants. The statistical analysis showed a whopping decline in LDL of 14 mg/dL with regular psyllium consumption. The researchers believe that this decreases the risk of a cardiovascular event, such as a heart attack or stroke, by 7 percent.

The scientists explain that psyllium works to lower LDL cholesterol in two main ways. First, the soluble fiber in psyllium helps your body break down cholesterol more effectively. It also helps your liver create more "docking stations" (called LDL receptors) that grab on to bad cholesterol floating in your bloodstream and remove it. Second, when you eat psyllium, the fiber travels to your gut, where it undergoes fermentation (see "Fermentability, Another Virtue of Soluble Fiber," page 102).

In simple terms: psyllium fiber helps your body both get rid of existing LDL cholesterol and use up cholesterol stores, giving you a double benefit for heart health.

Source: Z. Ruiting et al., "Plantago Consumption Significantly Reduces Total Cholesterol and Low-Density Lipoprotein Cholesterol in Adults: A Systematic Review and Meta-Analysis," *Nutrition Research* 126 (June 2024): 123–137.

Method of Attack #2. Soluble fiber helps keep cholesterol and fat from entering intestinal cells. It does this by expanding the unstirred water layer, which increases the barrier for diffusion of fat and cholesterol and disturbs the formation of micelles (the cholesterol transport vehicles). This, in turn, alters the liver's concentration of cholesterol and fat.

Why does this matter in the context of LDL cholesterol reduction? Just as we saw with the soluble fiber in flaxseeds, psyllium works to reduce LDL by first affecting the VLDL particle makeup. Recall from Chapter 1 that VLDL is made in the liver and is the parent of LDL. In a study of psyllium-fed guinea pigs, scientists found that psyllium intake resulted in less intestinal absorption of cholesterol and fat, the building blocks of the VLDL molecule.[11] Thus, psyllium intake modified the nature, size, and composition of the VLDL particles. These beneficial compositional changes translate into a reduction in the amount of LDL formed from VLDL, and LDL and VLDL particles are more likely to be sucked back into receptors on the liver cells, leading to an overall reduction in "bad" cholesterol.

Method of Attack #3. Another LDL-lowering tactic is related to two key cholesterol metabolism enzymes: HMG-CoA reductase and 7 alpha-hydroxylase. HMG-CoA reductase is the main enzyme in the liver cell's cholesterol production pathway, whereas 7 alpha-hydroxylase is the regulating enzyme in the production of bile acids from cholesterol. Soluble fiber stymies the activity of HMG-CoA reductase and increases the activity of 7 alpha-hydroxylase.[12] Decreased HMG-CoA reductase activity means less cholesterol produced by liver cells. Stimulation of 7 alpha-hydroxylase increases bile acid production from cholesterol. Both scenarios lead to less internal cholesterol and increased clearance of LDL from the bloodstream.

Method of Attack #4. Psyllium also lowers LDL cholesterol by cordoning off glucose, resulting in reduced glucose uptake by the cells lining the small intestine, which in turn lowers insulin levels. This curtails the activity of the main cholesterol-manufacturing enzyme, HMG-CoA reductase, which, as we have learned, means less cholesterol supply in liver cells, a factor that leads to increased clearance of LDL from the bloodstream to compensate.

Should I Take Metamucil Plus Calcium Capsules?

To ensure good health and in particular good bone health, men and women should aim for a dietary intake of 1,000 mg of calcium per day (age fifty and under) and 1,200 mg per day (over age fifty). If you are not getting the recommended amount of calcium from food (and most Americans are not), then by all means add in calcium supplements.

If you choose to take Metamucil capsules with added calcium, you should know that each capsule contains *less* psyllium husk than the regular Metamucil capsules (0.42 grams vs. 0.52 grams).

Therefore, to reach the Cholesterol Down starting daily goal of 3 grams of psyllium husk per day, you would need to take seven Metamucil Plus Calcium capsules (supplying about 300 mg of calcium). To reach the most therapeutic goal of 10 grams of psyllium husk per day, you would need to take 24 capsules (supplying about 1,000 mg calcium). As this might not be the most practical idea, I suggest sticking with either the regular Metamucil capsules (or two servings per day of Metamucil powder) and adding in a separate calcium supplement.

PSYLLIUM CAUTION

Several caveats exist regarding Metamucil supplements. Fiber supplements and high-fiber foods can sometimes result in gas and bloating, but you can avoid these unpleasant side effects if you start with a low dose of fiber and gradually increase it over time. I would suggest that you begin by taking no more than 3 grams of psyllium husk per day (about six Metamucil capsules or one serving of Metamucil powder) and see how your body handles the fiber from the supplements in addition to all the other sources of fiber in the Cholesterol Down Plan. Gradually work your way up to the full prescription, allowing your system to adjust. If you take the capsules, be sure to swallow them with a *full glass or two of water* to ensure that they flow completely down the throat. You should also be aware that there have been reports in the literature, albeit rare, of severe allergic reactions to psyllium. Check with your doctor first before adding this step into your Cholesterol Down routine.

FILLING THE PRESCRIPTION

To consume the Cholesterol Down daily goal of 12 grams of soluble fiber, several servings of a psyllium fiber supplement will get you almost half of your daily dose in the form of psyllium. After you have successfully experimented with one serving, divide your daily dose in two so that you can take one half in the morning before breakfast and the other half after dinner.

If capsules are not the method you prefer for getting in your psyllium, Metamucil offers additional psyllium-containing products. If you can afford the calories, try Metamucil's crispy wafers in apple and cinnamon flavor. Two wafers total about 3 grams of psyllium husk. Or you can take Metamucil the old-fashioned way, in powder form (1 serving provides 2.4 grams of soluble fiber from psyllium husk). Note that consuming 10 grams of psyllium husk provides approximately 7 grams of viscous soluble fiber.

Metamucil offers a wide range of products, but not all Metamucil products contain psyllium husk. For example, Metamucil gummies contain inulin as the fiber source, not psyllium! There are also numerous additional companies (such as GNC, Nature's Herbs, Nature's Way, Solgar, and Yerba Prima) that sell psyllium husk products, and any of those products would also suffice for the Cholesterol Down Plan. All Star Health has a product list for psyllium husk on its website (www.allstarhealth.com). Countless fiber supplements crowd store shelves, each promising digestive benefits. When choosing one, examine the ingredients carefully—psyllium seed husk should top the ingredient list as the primary component. Just make sure to scrutinize the label and aim for a starting dose of about 3 grams per day of psyllium husk, building up to about 7 to 10 grams per day.

Psyllium Product	Amount	Psyllium Seed Husk
Metamucil wafers	2 wafers (120 calories)	3.0 grams
Metamucil powder	1 rounded tablespoon or 1 rounded teaspoon (depending on product) (about 45 calories)	3.4 grams
Metamucil supplements	1 capsule (10 calories for 6 capsules)	0.52 grams
Metamucil Plus Calcium supplements	1 capsule (10 calories for 5 capsules)	0.42 grams
Country Life psyllium seed husk capsules	3 capsules (5 calories)	1.5 grams
Yerba Prima psyllium husks capsules	4 capsules (8 calories)	2.2 grams
Nature's Way psyllium husk capsules	6 capsules (10 calories)	3.15 grams
Now Foods psyllium husk capsules (500 mg)	3 capsules (5 calories)	1.5 grams
GNC psyllium seed husk capsules (500 mg)	1 capsule (no calories listed on the Nutrition Facts label)	0.5 grams
Puritan's Pride psyllium husk capsules (750 mg)	2 capsules (no calories listed on the Nutrition Facts label)	1.5 grams

Psyllium Husks and Fiber on the Internet

For more information on psyllium husk supplement and fiber, log on to the following websites.

American Heart Association (www.heart.org/en/healthy-living/healthy-eating/eat-smart/nutrition-basics/whole-grains-refined-grains-and-dietary-fiber)

Harvard Health Publishing (www.health.harvard.edu/heart-health/psyllium-fiber-regularity-and-healthier-lipid-levels)

FDA Consumer Information (www.fda.gov/food/nutrition-food-labeling-and-critical-foods/authorized-health-claims-meet-significant-scientific-agreement-ssa-standard)

Health Canada (Psyllium and Cholesterol) (www.canada.ca/en/health-canada/services/food-nutrition/food-labelling/health-claims/assessments/psyllium-products-blood-cholesterol-lowering-nutrition-health-claims-food-labelling.html)

FH Australasia Network (www.athero.org.au/fh/patients/treatment-lifestyle/healthy-diet/psyllium/)

CHAPTER 8

Step 5: Eat Beans

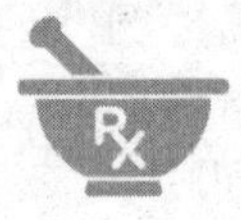

Eat ½ cup of legumes (beans, peas, or lentils) every day.

"I have trouble adding beans into my diet. Do you have any suggestions on how I can get them in?" That's a question I have been asked by some of my patients. My response is "However you can manage it, try to get some kind of beans in, as they are about as good as it gets for a healthy protein source. Try ordering a bean burrito 'Fresco style' at Taco Bell (they'll leave out the dairy and some egg-based items and replace them with diced tomatoes). You can ask for minestrone soup at your local Italian restaurant or even carry a to-go container of vegetarian baked beans with you for a sweet snack if you are on the go."

THE BENEFITS OF EATING BEANS

Beans, peas, and lentils are categorized as both part of the vegetable and the protein foods groups in the USDA's MyPlate dietary guidelines, making beans extraordinarily versatile. Not only are beans an excellent source of fiber (both soluble and insoluble), they are economical warehouses of plant protein and virtually fat-free, which should make them the number one protein source for heart-health-conscious individuals.

What's more, unlike meat, beans are free of saturated fat and cholesterol and extremely inexpensive. It doesn't get much better than that.

Tom's Story

Thomas D., age forty-five

Pre: Total cholesterol: 246 mg/dL; LDL cholesterol: 168 mg/dL

Post: Total cholesterol: 198 mg/dL; LDL cholesterol: 125 mg/dL

26 percent reduction in LDL cholesterol

Tom is the driven, highly successful president of an insurance agency and real estate corporation and is married with one daughter. His discipline and strong work ethic also apply to his healthy lifestyle choices: he eats a balanced diet and is in top physical condition. Despite this, Tom has always battled a genetic tendency toward high cholesterol. Concerned about Tom's elevated cholesterol, yet unwilling to start him on a statin without first trying lifestyle changes, Tom's physician referred him to me. Tom describes his experience with the Cholesterol Down Plan.

I have always exercised since I was a child. When I was in my teens, I started fighting in kickboxing tournaments. I always had a trainer who watched my diet. Sometimes I had to gain weight, sometimes I had to lose, depending on my weight class. I never had a problem with my cholesterol until I was in my late thirties or early forties. I don't know much about my family history since I lost my parents when I was very young, but I know that my sister also has high cholesterol. Recently, during a routine physical exam, I learned that my total cholesterol was higher than ever before at 246 mg/dL. I was a little concerned. My doctor suggested that I try lifestyle and diet changes to get my cholesterol under control and introduced me to a nutritionist—Dr. Janet Brill.

I went on Dr. Brill's special diet for thirty days. I really didn't have to take away the foods I enjoyed, I just had to add some important nutrients to my diet. I added soy, fiber, and some nutritional supplements, and I made a few substitutions. It was very easy to follow, and I actually enjoyed it. After thirty days, I had my cholesterol retested, and the results were amazing! My total cholesterol dropped to the lowest it has ever been, 198. I lowered my LDL to 125, and my HDL remained steady. I even lost a few pounds in the process, and I am starting to see more definition in my abs.

Dr. Brill's diet is the best I have ever tried. It was delicious and satisfying, and I have much more energy. I feel like I'm in my twenties again. Dr. Brill is the best nutritionist I have ever worked with. In my opinion, she is truly a miracle worker.

All beans are similar in terms of nutritional makeup, loaded with the minerals iron, zinc, calcium, magnesium, and potassium as well as the B vitamins thiamin, riboflavin, folate, and niacin. Potassium and magnesium are especially heart-friendly minerals that keep blood pressure in check. Beans are one of the plant kingdom's greatest sources of folate, a water-soluble B vitamin necessary for preventing birth defects in addition to contributing to heart health. And that's not all. Beans are packed with throngs of disease-fighting phytochemicals and antioxidants. The fact that beans are virtual vats of complex carbohydrates makes them a high-energy food, ideal for promoting an even flow of glucose (sugar) into the bloodstream.

It is not an exaggeration to say that beans are the superstars of health food. Not only does consuming beans reduce risk of heart disease, but beans also do the following:

- Help control diabetes by regulating blood sugar
- Battle obesity by moderating hunger
- Lower the risk of different types of cancer (lung, colon, breast, esophagus, and stomach) by virtue of their fiber and antioxidant composition

- Help prevent unpleasant digestive system ills such as constipation and hemorrhoids
- increase longevity[1]

BEANS, BEANS, GOOD FOR YOUR HEART

No doubt about it, eating legumes—beans, peas, lentils—is good for the heart. Eat them four times or more per week, and you could cut your risk of heart disease by an astounding 22 percent, as shown in a nineteen-year study of more than 10,000 American men and women published in the highly esteemed journal *Archives of Internal Medicine.*[2]

BEANS CUT CHOLESTEROL

Eating lots of legumes protects you against heart disease by making a huge dent in your "bad" cholesterol level. In fact, beans are just as effective in cutting LDL as that old cholesterol-lowering staple, oat bran. A study comparing the impact of supplementing diets of people with high cholesterol with either ingredient showed oat bran (3.5 ounces per day) lowered LDL by 23 percent and either navy or pinto beans (¾ cup per day) by 24 percent after a mere twenty-one days.[3] Further scientific evidence for the cholesterol-lowering power of beans comes from a meta-analysis published in the *British Journal of Nutrition,* in which eleven clinical studies concluded that eating legumes other than soybeans lowers LDL cholesterol by 7 percent in individuals with high initial cholesterol levels.[4] A more recent randomized trial confirmed that eating a cup of beans every day for 4 weeks lowered LDL by 8 percent.[5]

WHAT IS IT IN BEANS THAT LOWERS CHOLESTEROL?

Of all the prescribed foods in the Cholesterol Down Plan, beans lead the pack in terms of soluble fiber content. The science supports the notion that the greater your intake of soluble fiber, the larger the decrease in LDL cholesterol. Unlike the soluble fiber in psyllium, bean fiber does not increase the amount of bile acids excreted (one mechanism of lowering LDL is to increase bile acids out of the body). So, if that's not it, how do beans fight LDL and protect the heart?

Method of Attack #1. Scientists at the University of Kentucky think the key cholesterol-lowering mechanism lies in bean fiber's ability to be fermented in the colon, like psyllium.[6] Healthful bacteria feast on both beans' soluble fibers and innate sugars to generate short-chain fatty acids, which then hinder cholesterol production in the liver. Thus beans are considered important prebiotics for promoting both colon and heart health.

Method of Attack #2. As noted previously, beans are loaded with soluble fiber. One way that the soluble fiber in beans works to lower LDL is by altering cholesterol diffusion dynamics within the intestine. Beans speed transit time within the intestine, which lowers the rate of cholesterol absorption. What's more, beans can increase the bulk of the intestinal contents, which can widen the unstirred water layer, making it even more difficult for cholesterol to cross into the intestinal cells. The end result is a depletion of the cholesterol pool in liver cells. Thus, scientists have stated that the major method by which soluble fiber lowers blood cholesterol is through an increase in the number of LDL receptors to compensate for depleted liver cholesterol stores.[7] More receptors equate to greater LDL clearance from the bloodstream.

Method of Attack #3. Beans slow absorption of glucose into the bloodstream, decreasing the amount of insulin released from the pancreas. Insulin stimulates liver production of lipoproteins, so less insulin means less VLDL pumped out.

Method of Attack #4. Studies suggest that a component of several species of legumes (a protein chain called 7S globulin) can increase liver LDL and beta-VLDL receptor activity, therefore decreasing LDL in the bloodstream. In addition, beans, peas, and lentils have amino acid profiles similar to soy protein, oats, and almonds, all of which are rich in an amino acid called arginine. As discussed in Chapter 11, arginine keeps blood vessels relaxed and expanded, to help prevent atherosclerosis.

Method of Attack #5. Besides supplying healthy plant protein, beans also contain an array of phytochemicals, powerful chemicals that can squelch plaque buildup by dismantling the free radicals that oxidize LDL during the process of atherosclerosis.

BEANS . . . THEY'RE A REAL GAS

Never fails. I put beans on the dinner table and my nine-year-old happily recites the familiar schoolyard chant: "Beans, beans, they're good for your heart, the more you eat, the more you—" Well, you get the picture! Raffinose is the notorious sugar-like compound in beans that is the most responsible for beans' reputation as being bad for your social life. Bacteria in the lower digestive tract digest the beans but have trouble with the raffinose and other sugars, releasing an assortment of gases in the process. Beans are not the only offenders. Other healthy foods such as cabbage, Brussels sprouts, broccoli, cauliflower, oat bran, and most of the heart-healthy foods high in soluble fiber also promote gas formation.

In general, the large amount of fiber in the Cholesterol Down Plan may cause some gas and bloating or even require more frequent trips to the bathroom—but this is perfectly normal and will abate with time. So, take heart. After a few weeks' time, your digestive system will adapt to bean consumption with noticeably less discomfort. If that's not consolation enough, the sidebar below lists six bean tips that will help cut down on the gas problem.

Six Tips to Help De-Gas Those Beans

1. Sprinkle a few drops of Beano (an enzyme preparation) on food according to package directions. Beano (www.beanogas.com from GlaxoSmithKline) helps relieve the gas and bloating some people experience when adding in unfamiliar high-fiber foods to the diet.

2. Cook beans thoroughly; skim and discard the foam off the top of the cooking water.
3. If you choose to soak your own beans rather than use canned, make sure to rinse the beans well and drain the soaking and cooking water. Never cook the beans in the soaking water or you defeat the purpose—use fresh liquid for a soup base.
4. Add beans *gradually* to your diet to allow your digestive tract to adjust to the high-fiber intake. Too much fiber too fast will have unpleasant side effects. Stick to the plan and adjust bean intake as necessary. Remember, your body needs some time to adapt.
5. Chew beans thoroughly and drink lots of fluids.
6. Exercise it off. Mild exercise, such as your daily Cholesterol Down walk (Chapter 13), helps speed the passage of gas through the intestine.

FILLING THE PRESCRIPTION

There are two broad categories of beans: fresh and dried. Fresh beans are generally sold in the form just picked from the garden. Familiar examples are green beans (eaten in their pod), fava beans (aka broad beans), and my childhood favorite, lima beans (also known as butter beans for their creamy texture). Note that green beans do not provide either the fiber or the nutrients available in other types of beans and should therefore not be counted toward filling your daily bean prescription. (Fava and lima beans, on the other hand, are chock-full of LDL-lowering soluble fiber—1.2 grams in ½ cup of fava beans and a whopping 3.5 grams in ½ cup of lima beans.) Dried beans, peas, and lentils are the mature dried seeds of legumes, picked from the vine only after the natural maturation process has been completed. The term "legumes" actually refers to both beans packaged in bags and precooked canned beans.

If you have the time and the energy, the superior taste of do-it-yourself beans is well worth the extra effort of sorting, soaking, rinsing, and cooking prepackaged dried beans. To soak or not to soak? It is not necessary to soak dried beans before cooking them. However, soaking has benefits; among other things it removes much of the gas-producing sugars that dissolve in the soaking water. Always rinse beans after soaking and discard the water to get rid of as much of these troublesome substances as possible. Second, soaking beans before cooking softens and rehydrates them. The "quick soak" method consists of tossing beans in boiling water, turning off the heat, and soaking them for at least an hour. The traditional soaking technique involves soaking a pound of dried beans in six cups of water overnight.

To speed things up, you can use a pressure cooker, which can drastically reduce the cooking time for dried beans, whether they have been soaked or not. You might also consider a slow cooker. Slow cookers can also cook dried beans without soaking, although the cooking time will be longer than with other methods.

For those who prefer the quickest and most convenient method of eating beans, use canned. Not to worry—you will still get all the bean nutrition. Just be sure to give them a quick rinse to get rid of most of the added sodium before use. Dried beans will stay good for up to twelve months when stored in an airtight container at room temperature. Canned beans should be used within one year of the stamped expiration date.

Whether you choose to soak and cook them yourself or take the easier canned route, beans are one of nature's top cholesterol-busting foods. They're healthy, inexpensive, and great-tasting, so be sure to make them a staple of your diet.

Five Tips for Adding Beans into Your Day

1. Eat at salad bars and add chickpeas or kidney beans to your plate.
2. Puree beans and use as a sandwich spread or dip.
3. Routinely serve beans as a side dish on your dinner plate, such as black beans and rice or baked beans.

4. Eat cultural foods that incorporate beans, such as Mexican and Latin American dishes.
5. Make soup with beans: split pea soup, lentil soup, etc.

There are myriad types of dried beans—at least fifty varieties, each with its own interesting historical and cultural ties. A few examples:

- **Adzuki beans** are common in Asian cuisine. Japanese often use them to make a sweet red bean paste.
- **Black beans** (aka turtle beans or frijoles negros) are native to South America and a staple of Latin cuisine and delectable Caribbean-style dishes.
- **Black-eyed peas** (pea beans) have a long history from China and the Silk Road to traditional southern dishes derived from plantation cooking.
- **Cannellini beans** are those small white beans often showcased in Italian fare such as delicious Tuscan white bean soup.
- **Chickpeas** (garbanzo beans) are used to make the Middle Eastern favorite hummus, among other things.
- **Kidney beans** are so named for their resemblance to the shape of our organs. They are indigenous to southwestern dishes such as chili.
- **Lentils** are the easiest to cook, as they do not require soaking first. What's more, they are the legume highest in folate and fiber. Lentils are a staple in the spicy East Indian dishes known as dals. Lentils are so common in India that it is said every house there cooks them in one form or another almost every day.
- **Pinto beans** (from the Spanish word for "painted," as they resemble the horse of the same name) may be most familiar to you for their use in Mexican-style dishes such as burritos and refried beans.
- **Navy beans** have historical significance. They were named for their use in the thick and creamy white soups that

nourished U.S. naval forces during World War II. They are also used today to make Boston's well-known baked beans.

- **Split peas** are just that. Their hull is split into two halves, most often used to make the warm and savory classic split pea soup.

Bean Product	Fiber	Total Amount	Soluble Fiber
Canned beans, drained and rinsed	½ cup (100 calories)	7 grams	3 grams
Dried beans, peas, lentils	½ cup cooked (100 calories)	7 grams	3 grams

Beans on the Internet

For everything you ever wanted to know about beans, plus many delicious bean recipes, please refer to the following websites.

U.S. Dry Bean Council (https://usdrybeans.com)
Michigan Bean Commission (https://michiganbean.com)
Central Bean Company (www.centralbean.com)
Bush Brothers and Company (www.bushbeans.com)
American Heart Association (www.heart.org/en/healthy-living/healthy-eating/eat-smart/nutrition-basics/the-benefits-of-beans-and-legumes)

CHAPTER 9

Step 6: Eat Apples

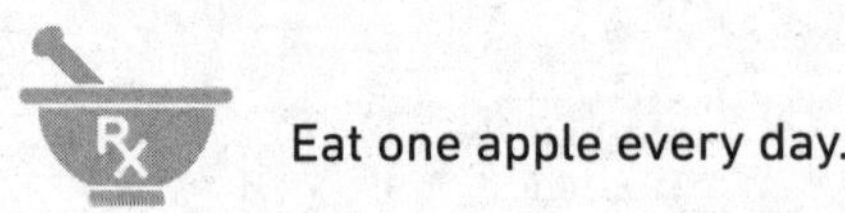

Eat one apple every day.

An older male patient of mine who had been on a statin drug for years once said to me, "I take pectin supplements to lower my cholesterol, so why should I eat apples?" Apples contain a wealth of cholesterol-fighting compounds, most notably pectin, but also many antioxidants and dietary fiber. In addition to lowering cholesterol, they have been shown to reduce the risk of lung and prostate cancer, all while providing these health benefits:

- The pectin in apples helps diabetics maintain a steady blood sugar level.
- Apples are an excellent addition to any weight loss plan. Low-calorie and nutrient-dense, they are a filling and portable sweet treat, ideal for curbing hunger pangs.
- Apples are helpful in maintaining healthy lung function and have even been shown to ameliorate asthma symptoms.
- Called "nature's toothbrush," apples work the gums and clean the teeth.
- The tannins in apples help to ward off urinary tract infections.

Charles's Story

Charles D., age fifty-seven

Pre: Total cholesterol: 305 mg/dL; LDL cholesterol: 182 mg/dL

Post: Total cholesterol: 223 mg/dL; LDL cholesterol: 124 mg/dL

32 percent reduction in LDL cholesterol

Charles is a highly successful dealer of antiques and collectibles. Though his health is generally good, he has several major risk factors for heart disease: he is a male over the age of forty-five; he has a strong family history of heart disease; he lives with overweight; and his LDL cholesterol is dangerously high. Charles has been taking Mevacor (20 mg) to control his high cholesterol and has experienced no side effects. However, medication alone has not been sufficient to reduce his cholesterol to the desired level. Fully aware of his high-risk status, he decided to seek my help. Here is what Charles has to say about his experience with the Cholesterol Down Plan.

Dr. Brill's program is very easy to stick with, as all the items are simple to find—in fact, most were available at my local supermarket—and also were very palatable. I chose to get the Metamucil step in by eating the Metamucil cookies instead of using the pills or powder, and I found them to be quite tasty and easy to carry around. The butter substitute (Take Control margarine) tastes good, and so it was easy to add into my daily diet as well. Spaced out over the whole day, nothing on the program really got boring.

I am sure I will be able to stick to the Cholesterol Down Plan over the long term. The walking was very manageable for me, as I play golf quite a few times a week and now enjoy walking the course instead of taking the cart. I am very glad that Dr. Brill was recommended to me by a friend. My results were obviously very satisfying to see. Thank you, Dr. Brill.

CAN I DRINK APPLE JUICE INSTEAD?

Nutritionists cringe at questions such as this and will always recommend that individuals eat the whole food instead of drinking the juice. Here's why.

1. One 8-ounce glass of apple juice contains roughly 117 calories, whereas one small apple contains approximately 55 calories.
2. The whole fruit takes longer to chew and is more filling, as it contains almost 5 grams of fiber; in contrast, the juice is devoid of fiber and many of the other healthful nutrients found in the whole fruit.
3. For weight control, "try not to drink your calories" is advice I give my patients. This is because it is just too easy to swallow hundreds of liquid calories in a matter of minutes compared to the longer and much more satisfying process of eating the whole fruit, which contains considerably fewer calories. If you opt for getting your fruits and vegetables in a liquid beverage rather than in solid form, I recommend tossing them in a blender rather than a juicer. Most juicers extract the pulp (fiber), leaving only a fraction of the healthful pectin.
4. For cholesterol lowering, it is the fiber and invisible phytochemicals concentrated in the discarded skin and pulp that are most important.

PECTIN LOWERS BAD CHOLESTEROL

As you learned in previous chapters, fiber comes in many forms. Several of the steps in the Cholesterol Down Plan involve foods or supplements that are high in gums and mucilage (flaxseeds, psyllium, and beans) and beta-glucan (oats and barley)—all different types of soluble, or viscous, fiber. Pectin is another type of soluble fiber, highly viscous in nature, and thus able to lower LDL cholesterol.

Pectin in apples changes from a water-insoluble substance when the fruit is green to the more water-soluble form in ripened fruit. Once digested, mature pectin, like other types of soluble fiber, forms a thick gel-like matter within the intestine. Like other fermentable fibers, once pectin reaches the colon, it is consumed by friendly bacteria to release short-chain fatty acids, primarily acetate. Acetate may promote cardiovascular health by making the blood less likely to clot.

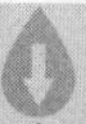

Two Apples a Day Magnify LDL Reduction

If you love apples, great news! A randomized, controlled intervention study has proven that consuming two apples a day instead of one results in dramatic reductions in LDL. Forty healthy men and women ate two fresh, whole apples a day for a period of 8 weeks. At the end of the study, the apple eaters had an average drop in LDL of 14 mg/dL The researchers state that apple polyphenols play a major role in lowering cholesterol and work synergistically with the pectin/soluble fiber in apples to produce these impressive results.

Source: A. Koutsos et al., "Two Apples a Day Lower Serum Cholesterol and Improve Cardiometabolic Biomarkers in Mildly Hypercholesterolemic Adults: A Randomized, Controlled, Crossover Trial." *American Journal of Clinical Nutrition* 111 (2020): 307–318.

WHY EAT PECTIN IF YOU'RE ALREADY CONSUMING BETA-GLUCAN AND PSYLLIUM?

Each specific source of soluble fiber is associated with both similar and distinctly different mechanisms of action for lowering LDL cholesterol. When scientists at the University of Arizona in Tucson experimented with guinea pigs that had been fed one of three types of soluble fiber—psyllium, pectin, or guar gum—and compared them to a control group fed the insoluble fiber cellulose, the scientists found that all sources of soluble fiber reduced LDL cholesterol (with no cholesterol-lowering effect observed in the cellulose-fed animals).[1] The researchers also observed that the different types of soluble fibers had decidedly different cholesterol-lowering mechanisms, specific to each fiber. This study provides further scientific support for the Cholesterol Down daily recommendation to consume a diverse assortment of foods containing different types of soluble fiber.

HOW PECTIN AND PSYLLIUM COMPARE

Soluble fibers work in the intestine to cut cholesterol in two ways: by slowing the recycling of bile acids and by decreasing cholesterol absorption. Both psyllium and pectin are viscous gel-forming fibers that bind up bile acids, resulting in slowed bile acid recycling and greater excretion in the stool. The resulting shortage of bile acids returning to the liver forces the liver to use its cholesterol supply to make new bile acids—and to replenish supplies by sucking up more LDL from the bloodstream. Pectin is also similar to psyllium in that it prevents absorption of cholesterol from the intestine. This translates into less cholesterol returning to the liver, reduced production of VLDL, and consequently lower blood LDL.

How do pectin and psyllium differ in their cholesterol-lowering methods? A study in guinea pigs (guinea pigs have a cholesterol response to fiber similar to humans) set out to answer this question.[2] It turns out that the difference lies in how each fiber affects the makeup of the nascent VLDL particles produced by the liver. Researchers discerned that pectin affects the composition of the VLDL particle by enriching it with much more fat (triglycerides). This leads to fewer and more fat-filled VLDLs released from the liver. Plus, the composition of these particles makes them much more likely to be broken down by fat-burning enzymes. Since VLDL is the precursor of LDL, less VLDL secreted means less LDL formed in the blood. Psyllium, on the other hand, changes the VLDL makeup such that there is much less esterified cholesterol and more phospholipids. Once released from the liver into the bloodstream, this transformed VLDL particle is less able to be converted to LDL and is more readily removed from the bloodstream via LDL and beta-VLDL receptors, thus it is a different mechanism for reducing LDL. The main point with regard to apple pectin is that it lowers LDL in ways both similar to and different from psyllium, so by combining both steps, you get a much stronger cholesterol-lowering effect.

What about pectin in humans? A large study of middle-aged men and women living in the Los Angeles area assessed the relationship between intake of this particular dietary fiber and the progression of atherosclerosis.[3] Five hundred individuals gave detailed dietary information and had their carotid arteries (neck arteries leading to the brain) examined for evidence of atherosclerosis. The higher the intake of pectin in the diet, the less atherosclerotic plaque that was evident in the carotid arteries, suggesting a slowing of the atherosclerotic process. A more recent trial[4] looked at the effects of eating an apple a day in 250 study participants for a period of 4 months. Four groups were administered one apple per day among the following: Red Delicious, Granny Smith, Fuji, Golden Delicious. The fifth group was asked to consume two Annurca apples per day. Comparing results, the two-apple-a-day group reduced LDL cholesterol by a phenomenal 14.5 percent and increased high-density lipoprotein cholesterol level by 15.2 percent.

THE ANTIOXIDANT CONNECTION

What protection does your body have against attack by disease-causing free radicals? The answer is antioxidants, otherwise known as free radical scavengers. Unstable oxygen free radical molecules are created through normal cellular metabolism. Excessive amounts are formed through exposure to radiation and pollution. The body uses antioxidants to stop free radicals before they start a chain reaction of oxidation that damages cells and DNA and can eventually lead to atherosclerosis. How do you boost your antioxidant army? Eat lots of fruits and vegetables, which contain hundreds if not thousands of different types of antioxidants. You are probably already familiar with some of the best-known antioxidant vitamins and minerals: vitamin C, vitamin E, selenium, and beta-carotene. In addition, apples are packed with polyphenols, a special type of plant antioxidant linked to reduced risk of chronic disease, including cardiovascular disease.

When It Comes to Antioxidants, All Apples Are Not Created Equal

Apples contain a virtual cocktail of antioxidants, possibly thousands of plant chemicals that all work together to deliver the significant health benefits linked with the whole fruit. We know that the antioxidant activity seen with apples is way more than vitamin C, an antioxidant vitamin, is able to confer alone.

A Canadian government study analyzed eight different varieties of apples (Red Delicious, Northern Spy, McIntosh, Cortland, Ida Red, Golden Delicious, Mutsu, and Empire) for their antioxidant content. Red Delicious apples had several hundred times the antioxidant activity that scientists would have expected from their vitamin C content alone. In fact, of the eight varieties analyzed, Red Delicious, the most commonly grown apple in the United States, and another type, Northern Spy, had the highest concentration of antioxidants. Another analysis of ten varieties of apples commonly eaten in the United States showed that Fuji, Red Delicious, Gala, and Liberty apples lead the pack in terms of healthful phenolic acid content.

Sources: Rong Tsao et al., "Which Polyphenolic Compounds Contribute to the Total Antioxidant Activities of Apples?," *Journal of Agricultural and Food Chemistry* 53, no. 12 (2005): 4989–4995; Jeanelle Boyer and Rui Hai Liu, "Apple Phytochemicals and Their Health Benefits," *Nutrition Journal* 3 (2004), www.nutritionj.com/content/3/1/5.

STUDIES SHOW THAT APPLES CUT LDL CHOLESTEROL

Apples Resist Oxidation of LDL in Humans

Scientists out of the University of California at Davis showed the apple's power over LDL cholesterol.[5] They discovered that people eating two apples a day or drinking an equivalent amount of apple juice had a significant slowing of LDL oxidation, the process that results in plaque buildup. How do apples work to alter LDL metabolism?

Method of Attack #1. The scientists propose that the apple antioxidants are incorporated into the LDL molecule, so the antioxidant is oxidized in place of the LDL, preventing harm to the LDL molecule and thus helping to impede the progression of atherosclerosis.

Method of Attack #2. A doctoral student at Cornell University performed test-tube experiments showing that not only can an extract of Red Delicious apples prevent the oxidation of human LDL cholesterol, but the extract also prompts the liver to sprout more LDL receptors, thereby reducing LDL levels in the bloodstream. Furthermore, apple extract dampens the activity of a key protein in liver cells that functions to signal the start of the cholesterol production pathway (termed the sterol regulatory element binding protein, or SREBP). Apples therefore work to squelch cholesterol production in a manner similar to statin drugs.[6]

APPLES CUT LDL BY 70 PERCENT, AT LEAST IN FAT RATS

It's a huge leap from rats to humans, but the results of one study are nonetheless eye-opening.[7] French scientists gave rats with obesity and high cholesterol an "apple diet" of regular rat chow plus ground-up apples for three weeks. It turns out the apple diet cut LDL cholesterol by a whopping 70 percent. How did apples lower LDL to this extent?

Method of Attack #3. The scientists noted a marked increase in the pool of bile acids in the intestines of the apple-fed rats compared to rats fed the control diet. Bile acids are formed in the liver from cholesterol. The increased amount of bile acids entering the intestine suggests the liver is working overtime to make new bile acids (requiring more cholesterol). This process results in less circulating LDL. Why would the liver increase its production of bile acids? The answer: less cholesterol is returning to the liver, as the recycling of bile acids is hindered by the apple diet.

The study authors suggested that the remarkable LDL-cutting ability of apples stemmed from the cholesterol-lowering effect of soluble fibers, primarily pectin, working together with the apple's polyphenol compounds to trap bile acids in the intestine. This is the same mechanism bile acid sequestrant drugs such as Questran use to lower LDL cholesterol.

Which of the compounds in apples is more effective at reducing LDL cholesterol, the pectin or the polyphenols? Another group of French researchers fed rats with high cholesterol a typical rat chow with one of three different additives: isolated apple pectin, isolated apple polyphenols, or a more natural apple combination of both pectin and polyphenols.[8] The natural combination additive of apple pectin and polyphenols was much more effective in lowering cholesterol than the isolated nutrients, suggesting that the interaction of the two components is best for maximum cholesterol reduction.

In addition, this same study noted that the antioxidant effects of the many polyphenols found in apples protect against heart disease by countering oxygen's damaging effects on cells and by preventing oxidation of LDL, an early step in cholesterol-filled plaque buildup. Thus, apple polyphenols reduce inflammation to decrease the risk of atherosclerosis in several ways.

POLYPHENOLS CUT LDL CHOLESTEROL

Method of Attack #4. Like many of the other foods in the Cholesterol Down Plan, the polyphenols in apples lower cholesterol absorption by interfering with cholesterol's ability to cross over from the small intestine into the intestinal cells. This disruption of cholesterol transport to the liver lowers the return rate of cholesterol. To compensate for this deficit, liver cells "turn on" more liver LDL receptors, resulting in a greater number of LDL particles being cleared from the bloodstream.[9]

Don't Toss the Peel!

It is best to eat the whole apple, peel and all, because a significant amount of polyphenols are located in the outer portion of the flesh and peel. The peel has more than six times the antioxidant activity of the flesh—another reason not to skimp on the skin (the potent polyphenol antioxidant quercetin is the main ingredient of apple peels). Furthermore, the peel contains about 1 gram of fiber and half the vitamin C content of the entire fruit.

Source: Rong Tsao et al., "Which Polyphenolic Compounds Contribute to the Total Antioxidant Activities of Apples?," *Journal of Agricultural and Food Chemistry* 53, no. 12 (2005): 4989–4995.

Method of Attack #5. Apple polyphenols affect the liver's construction of VLDL, the parent molecule of LDL, by modifying VLDL's packaging. Just like LDL, VLDL consists of an inner core of cholesterol and triglycerides, the entire particle encircled by a strand of protein called Apo B (VLDL has two additional proteins, Apo C and Apo E). Polyphenols interfere with the enzymes involved in the production of both of these core components (cholesterol and triglyceride), leading to a decline in their availability. Without enough of these core components, degradation of the Apo B protein occurs. These changes lead to less secretion of VLDL from the liver. The end result is lower blood levels of LDL.[10]

Method of Attack #6. Polyphenols found in apples have also been shown to positively affect blood vessel dynamics on several fronts. They reduce adhesion molecules, thus making the arterial wall less sticky and lowering the number of immune system blood cells that stick to the lining. This reduces inflammation and therefore helps protect against atherosclerosis. What's more, polyphenols reduce the ability of platelets to stick together, which lessens the ability of blood to clot, ultimately keeping a blood clot from choking off the blood supply to the heart muscle and thereby lowering your risk of a heart attack. Finally, polyphenols alter blood vessel mechanics by increasing the vessels' ability to relax and dilate. This also helps blood to flow more easily, reducing inflammation and risk of atherosclerosis.

APPLE CAUTION

Apples top the produce list when it comes to the highest level of pesticide residues, according to the Environmental Working Group, a not-for-profit environmental research organization. Two previous investigations list apples among the four most contaminated fruits, along with peaches, strawberries, and nectarines. In order to remove as much of the chemicals from the outer skin as possible, thoroughly rinse apples before eating them. Don't let the ads for spray products claiming to remove harmful pesticides fool you. While they may help to remove some of the surface pesticide residue, they do not eliminate them. In fact, a scientific study found that spray washes or detergents were no more effective in removing pesticide residues than rinsing thoroughly with tap water alone.[11]

The best way to avoid ingesting unacceptably high amounts of pesticides on a daily basis is to choose organically grown produce.

FILLING THE PRESCRIPTION

There are more than 2,500 different varieties of apples grown in the United States alone. Look for firm, shiny apples, blemish-free. Don't worry about the wax—ripe apples naturally develop a thin waxy coating to protect them from the elements. Much of this protective coat is lost during processing, so fruit purveyors add back a touch of FDA-approved, non-petroleum-based wax to keep those apples looking appetizing. Apples keep for an amazingly long period of time in your refrigerator bin, up to six months. Just be sure to throw out any apples with signs of decay, as they can accelerate aging in other apples in the bin. If cooking with apples, prevent browning of cut apples by keeping them in a bowl of ice water with a touch of lemon juice until ready to use in your recipe.

How Do You Like Them Apples?

If Red Delicious or Fuji apples (highest in antioxidants) are not your favorites, find one of the myriad apples on the market that you will enjoy eating on a daily basis. For baking, the Pippin, Granny Smith, Golden Delicious, Empire, and Jonagold varieties provide a great mix of sweetness and tartness when used in apple pie. Unless you are making baked apples or applesauce, avoid apples that get mushy when cooked, like McIntosh and Cortland.

Here is just a sampling of the many kinds of apples you may encounter at the supermarket—or, better yet, picked fresh off the tree.

- Braeburn apples originated down under (New Zealand), and with a rich, slightly tart flavor, they're perfect for snacking. They vary in color from an orangey yellow to red.
- Golden and Red Delicious are the thinnest-skinned apples. The familiar large and deeply colored Red Delicious is a classic and America's favorite snack apple, juicy and sweet without any hint of tartness. These types are extremely versatile, great for all-around use.
- Fuji apples (my personal favorite) are so named for their Japanese origin, Mount Fuji. Crisp, juicy, sweet, and perfect for that afternoon pick-me-up, these apples are colossal taste sensations.
- Jonagold is a hybrid of Jonathan apples and Golden Delicious bred in New York. A juicy apple with hints of orange color, this one is marvelous for making apple pie.

- Galas are the yellowish-orange-skinned apples with red stripes. Sweet and crisp, these apples are popular for snacking and in salads. Another apple with its origins in New Zealand, Galas are also a hybrid, a cross between Golden Delicious and Orange Pippin.

- Rome Beauty is the classic baking apple. Deep red in color with some yellow, this apple holds its shape well under heat, with a flavor that truly intensifies with cooking—a baker's dream.

- The lovely Pink Lady apple has a unique tangy yet sweet flavor. Originally bred in Australia, this lady gets her name from the bright pink color that she sports during the crisp fall weather.

- Granny Smiths are tart green apples, crisp, juicy, and delicious in salads—another apple that originated in Australia. And yes, there really was a Granny Smith (Maria Smith) who lived on a farm in Ryde, Australia, in the mid-1800s. She was the first to identify the seedling that bears her name.

- McIntoshes are the white-fleshed and thick red-skinned apples that many associate with the orchard. They are one of America's favorite snacking apples.

- Lady apples are the adorable miniature apples that are mostly green in color and tinged with red. These apples are often displayed around Thanksgiving. Moms, take note—kids love them!

Just can't seem to get another apple in? Try some alternative apple eating strategies for a refreshing change in your Cholesterol Down routine. Dried apple rings are available at the supermarket. Or try baking your apple with a touch of cinnamon for a tasty dessert. To really spruce up your daily dose, spread a gob of peanut butter—or, better yet, almond butter—on your apple slices for a delicious and nutritious snack.

Sources: "The Best Apples for Baking," Martha Stewart, accessed August 19, 2025, www.marthastewart.com/8016487/best-apple-varieties-for-baking; "Apple Varieties," Food Reference, accessed August 19, 2025, www.foodreference.com/html/artapples.html.

Apple Product	Total Amount	Soluble Fiber
Dried apple rings	1 cup (209 calories)	About 3 grams
Apple chips	1 ounce (140 calories)	About 1 gram
Apple	One medium with skin (70 calories)	About 0.5 grams
Earthbound Farm Sweet Organic Apple Slices	5 ounces (80 calories)	About 0.5 grams
Natural unsweetened applesauce	½ cup	1.3 grams
Apple butter fruit spread	1 tablespoon (29 calories)	Negligible

Apples on the Internet

For more information on apples and for some delicious apple recipes, I refer you to the following websites.

Washington State Apple Commission (waapple.org)

Gardener's Network (www.gardenersnet.com/fruit/apples/history.htm)

Maine Apples. (https://maineapples.org/apple-facts)

Cook's Thesaurus (www.foodsubs.com/Apples.html)

California Apple Commission (www.calapple.org/apple-facts.html)

CHAPTER 10

Step 7: Take Phytosterols

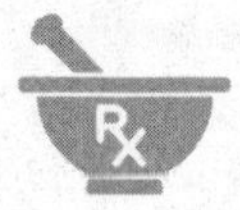

Consume 2–3 grams per day of phytosterols taken at two separate meals.

WHY EAT PHYTOSTEROLS (PLANT STEROLS AND STANOLS)?

Current guidelines[1] recommend Americans consume approximately 2 g/day plant sterols and plant stanols. This can reduce LDL cholesterol by approximately 10 percent when you combine this with other dietary changes. Phytosterols come in food form (such as in margarine) or in supplement form.

When I recommend to my patients that they add margarine to their diets, oftentimes their response is "I thought margarine is supposed to be worse for you than butter!" Others worry about margarine being an ultra-processed food—a valid concern that I'll address. Rest assured, butter is not good for the heart. It is a potent source of saturated fat, and saturated fat is one of the worst artery-clogging foods you can eat. Margarine, on the other hand, can be more healthful than butter because it is derived from polyunsaturated fat. While it's true that margarine is processed, certain varieties—particularly those enriched with plant sterols—offer proven cholesterol-lowering benefits that can outweigh these concerns for people managing their heart health. But don't just grab any type of margarine from the dairy shelf. Many brands of margarine, especially the stick types, are full of unhealthy saturated fat. Compare labels to find the spread with the least amount of saturated fat and sodium.

Roger's Story

Roger F., age fifty-nine

Pre: Total cholesterol: 215 mg/dL; LDL cholesterol: 105 mg/dL

Post: Total cholesterol: 162 mg/dL; LDL cholesterol: 69 mg/dL

34 percent reduction in LDL cholesterol

Roger is a middle-aged executive in good health and is overweight. He has been taking Lipitor (20 mg) for several years to control his high cholesterol and has experienced no side effects. Recently, his cardiologist became concerned about Roger's elevated cholesterol and triglyceride values and decided to increase Roger's Lipitor dosage to 40 mg per day. Not comfortable with the idea of doubling his statin dosage, Roger decided to give my diet a try. Here is Roger's account of his experience with the Cholesterol Down Plan.

I believe I am a fairly typical baby boomer who had been focused on family, career, and activities and had the opportunity of living overseas for many years. While aware of health issues (I have been fighting the battle of the bulge for a number of years), I was confused by the conflicting reports and claims regarding diets and healthy foods. Though I tried to "eat sensibly," I had a history of high cholesterol, and in 2000, when it reached 310, I was started on a statin drug that had immediate beneficial results. My cholesterol levels started to climb, and my doctor wanted me to increase my dosage of the statin drug, yet I was hesitant to increase the drug. Fortunately, I met Dr. Janet Brill and she put me on her LDL-lowering diet. The results were impressive, but best of all, the results were accomplished by eating a combination of foods that I was broadly familiar with and enjoyed. In fact, I was able to combine 80 percent of the daily food/supplement requirements in my breakfast oatmeal. This allowed significant flexibility for the rest of the day.

This is clearly a program that I can and will continue to follow. There was a definite period of adjustment for my system to handle the large increase in fiber. I did experience some bloating and at times didn't consume all of the daily requirements. Also, I found that I couldn't take the last dosage of soluble fiber close to bedtime; I had to allow at least three to four hours. But over time my system did become accustomed to the new diet, and the bloating subsided.

I am a total convert to this approach and am continuing it, with the goal of being able to eliminate the statin drugs completely.

Walk into any supermarket and you will most likely find "spreads" in the dairy section with labels boasting of their cholesterol-fighting abilities. This relatively new functional food is really a very tasty margarine-like concoction that happens to contain phytosterols, a safe and effective plant extract that can lower LDL cholesterol by an average of 10 percent without affecting your "good" HDL cholesterol in the process.

Choosing a Healthy Margarine

Smart Balance, I Can't Believe It's Not Butter, Earth Balance—with so many choices boasting of improved balance, smart choices, and better ratios, it's enough to make you just forget the whole thing and reach for the Land O'Lakes luscious butter (let's face it, nothing tastes as good as the real thing). So here are a few pointers on navigating the dairy case.

Rule 1: Look for margarines low in saturated fat. **The main culprit in raising LDL cholesterol is saturated fat, so select margarines with 2 grams or less per serving. Soft margarines (usually**

packaged in a tub) and liquid margarines tend to have less saturated fat and calories than stick margarines.

Rule 2: Check the ingredients list. Look for olive oil and canola oil at the beginning of the list. This means the spread has a higher amount of monounsaturated fatty acids and omega-3 polyunsaturated fatty acids, the heart-healthiest types.

Rule 3: Go for the "light" version. Margarines may be better for the heart but not so for the waistline. Regular tub margarines are still fat, and fat is a highly concentrated source of calories. Light versions of margarines (with added water) will reduce your calorie load.

Rule 4: Try plant-based spreads. Plant-based margarines provide a dairy-free substitute for butter, though their nutritional profiles vary considerably by brand and formulation. Most combine vegetable oils with water, salt, and fortifying nutrients such as vitamins A and D. What sets these spreads apart nutritionally is their reduced saturated fat content and complete absence of cholesterol—qualities that position them as a more heart-conscious choice than traditional butter.

Rule 5: Choose margarine with added phytosterols. Forget all the slick marketing campaigns about balance and heart health. *The heart-healthiest margarines contain phytosterols,* a scientifically proven means of cutting cholesterol. Read the fine print on the label and make sure the margarine you choose has some type of added phytosterol. Currently, the most readily available light margarine with added phytosterols is the Benecol Buttery Spread, Light brand.

FUNDAMENTALS OF PHYTOSTEROLS

What Exactly Are Phytosterols?

Phytosterols are found in the fat of plant foods and are basically the plant's version of cholesterol. Their structural similarity to human cholesterol is the basis for how they are able to lower LDL. Cholesterol is the primary sterol in humans. In plants as in humans, sterols are essential to life, functioning as building blocks for cell walls and steroid-based hormones. There are over forty different types of sterols found in plants. The National Cholesterol Education Program (NCEP) encourages Americans to consume between 2 and 3 grams per day of phytosterols to aid in cholesterol reduction.[2] Phytosterols have also been proven to protect against colon, breast, and prostate cancer.

FINDING PHYTOSTEROLS IN FOOD

There are two types of phytosterols: plant sterols, which are present naturally in vegetable oils, legumes, fruits, nuts, and seeds, and plant stanols, which are much less abundant in nature and contain added hydrogen. It is just not possible to eat enough plant foods in a day to receive the cholesterol-reducing dose of either, as the average American diet provides roughly 80 mg of phytosterols per day. Even a typical vegetarian diet, loaded with plant foods, contains only 300–400 mg of plant sterols and a small amount (25 mg) of plant stanols. This amount is way below the scientifically determined effective dosage of 2–3 grams per day shown to significantly reduce LDL cholesterol.

Therefore, the challenge for food scientists has been to invent a means of concentrating a large enough dose of phytosterols into an easily digestible and tasty product. This dilemma was solved by purifying and then modifying the naturally occurring phytosterols, most often derived from either soybean oil or tall oil, which comes from pine trees and other coniferous trees. After years of research, food scientists were successful in incorporating concentrated amounts into everyday foods, all capable of delivering a potent cholesterol-lowering punch. Different products contain different types of phytosterols, most with an added compound, or "esterified." Here are some examples:

- **Benecol margarine** was the first phytosterol-containing margarine on the U.S. market. Launched in Finland in 1995, it is now manufactured in the United States by the food giant McNeil, a division of Johnson & Johnson. Benecol contains a plant stanol derived from pine tree oil. The oil is a waste by-product obtained from trees during wood processing. In Benecol margarine, the stanol has a compound attached to it; hence you will see "plant stanol esters" on the label. Benecol also makes Soft Chews, a yummy chocolate treat that contains phytosterols. Four chews contain 2 grams of plant stanols, 80 calories, and 10 grams of sugar.

- **Promise Activ Light margarine** is manufactured by Lipton (parent company Unilever) and is enriched with a sterol derived from soybean oil. In this product, the plant sterol also has a compound attached to it, so you will find "plant sterol esters" written on this label.
- **Nature Made CholestOff supplements** have a form of plant sterols and stanols that have a compound attached to them, so you will find "plant sterol esters" written on the label. Note that there are 900 mg of phytosterols per serving (3 capsules) of CholestOff Complete and 900 mg of phytosterols per serving (2 capsules) of CholestOff Plus.

SHOW ME THE RESEARCH

Since the 1950s, plant sterols have been studied for their unique ability to lower cholesterol. The early studies used plant sterols in their free form (meaning not bound to any other compound).[3] These plant sterols were difficult to incorporate into food products because they dissolved too easily. They were also expensive and didn't taste very good. A resurgence of interest came about in the early 1990s, when a process known as esterification allowed for solubility in fatty products, such as mayonnaise. Now phytosterols can be found in everything from margarine to chewy gummy treats.

STUDIES PROVE PHYTOSTEROLS LOWER LDL CHOLESTEROL

In 1995, a landmark study on the dramatic LDL-lowering effect of phytosterol-enriched margarine was published in *The New England Journal of Medicine.*[4] The research was conducted in Finland, where 153 volunteers with high cholesterol were randomly divided into two groups. One group ate three servings (breakfast, lunch, and dinner) of regular margarine, and the other group consumed three servings of Benecol (providing a total of between 1.8 and 2.6 grams of a plant stanol ester per day). After one year, the Benecol group cut LDL by 14 percent compared to just 1 percent in the control group.

Confirming these results was another study out of Finland that tested the effect of three different kinds of spreads, as part of a low-fat diet, on the cholesterol level of thirty-four subjects.[5] The two phytosterol-containing spreads each contained a somewhat different stanol and sterol makeup, compared to the plain margarine, which did not contain any added phytosterols. Subjects ate their respective test margarine at each meal, such that the total daily phytosterol intake was approximately 2 grams for the two groups eating the test spreads. At the end of four weeks, LDL cholesterol dropped by 10 and 13 percent in the phytosterol margarine groups when compared to the control margarine group.

Another study supporting the significant cholesterol benefits of adding in a daily dose of margarine with phytosterols to a heart-healthy diet comes from the Chicago Center for Clinical Research.[6] Scientists divided 224 subjects with high cholesterol into three groups. All groups followed a traditional NCEP low-fat diet with their respective test margarine added into the diet. The three different test margarines were as follows: margarine containing a daily dose of either 1.1 grams (low-phytosterol group) or 2.2 grams (high-phytosterol group) of added phytosterols, or plain margarine. The margarines were eaten twice a day with other food. After just five weeks, the low-phytosterol margarine group lowered LDL cholesterol by 7 percent and the high-phytosterol group cut LDL by an impressive 10 percent compared to the control group. These findings suggest that eating the higher phytosterol dose of at least 2 grams per day (taken with food at two separate meals) is optimal for maximum LDL cholesterol lowering.

So strong was the scientific support for the cholesterol-lowering effect of phytosterols that their benefits were officially recognized by the FDA with a health claim in September 2000, which stated that foods containing plant stanol and sterols may reduce the risk of heart disease by lowering cholesterol. More than two decades later, the evidence has only grown stronger. In 2021, a review article published in the scientific journal *Nutrients* reaffirmed that phytosterol consumption remains a safe and highly effective strategy for lowering LDL cholesterol.[7] A panel of experts with diverse medical and scientific backgrounds convened by the Nutrition Foundation of Italy examined the accumulated research and concluded that phytosterols—whether as supplements or functional foods—can produce a 9–12.5 percent reduction in LDL cholesterol. The ideal dosage is 2–3 grams per day taken twice daily with food. This recent analysis not only validates the FDA's original position but also provides updated guidance for today's health professionals. The panel emphasized that phytosterols must be taken daily for continued benefit; while their cholesterol-lowering effect appears rapidly (within about three weeks), it is maintained only with routine intake.[8]

HOW DO PLANT STEROLS/STANOLS LOWER LDL CHOLESTEROL?

The 80 mg per day of phytosterols that the average person consumes from plant foods is too small to affect cholesterol metabolism. However, taken in doses of up to 3–4 grams per day, these plant chemicals lower LDL cholesterol by one key mechanism: blocking the absorption of dietary cholesterol and the resorption of bile cholesterol from the intestinal tract.

Method of Attack #1. Due to the similarity in chemical structure, phytosterols are able to masquerade as cholesterol, in effect blocking its absorption from the gut. Before it can gain entry into the intestinal cells, cholesterol must affix itself within an absorption vehicle called a micelle, but the phytosterols are more attracted to the limited spots on the micelle than the cholesterol. Phytosterols displace cholesterol and fool the body into granting it entry inside the intestinal cells instead. The result? Cholesterol absorption is decreased by about half, with a drop in both "bad" LDL and total cholesterol without affecting the level of "good" HDL cholesterol.

Interestingly, once inside the intestinal cells, plant sterols are not recognized by the human body and are returned back into the digestive tract and excreted with the rest of the solid waste.

Just how does blocked entry of intestinal cholesterol translate into lower amounts of LDL cholesterol circulating in the bloodstream? Less cholesterol returning from the intestine to the liver (via chylomicrons) triggers an increase in the number and the activity of LDL receptors. A greater number and more active receptors mean increased removal of LDL from the blood, by the liver, to restock the cholesterol supply. The overall effect is a lowering of blood LDL cholesterol.

WHAT'S THE RECOMMENDED PHYTOSTEROL INTAKE FOR CONTROLLING CHOLESTEROL?

Based on data from scores of scientific studies, the NCEP published a statement that reads: "Daily intakes of 2–3 grams per day of plant stanol/sterol esters will reduce LDL cholesterol by 6–15 percent. . . . Plant stanol/sterol esters (2 g/day) are a therapeutic option to enhance LDL cholesterol lowering."[9] The NCEP message is clear and concise: aim for consuming between 2 and 3 grams of plant sterol and/or stanol esters per day, divided between two meals, for maximum LDL cholesterol reduction.

Why divide your daily phytosterol dose between two meals instead of taking it just once a day? The bulk of the scientific research has shown that dividing the dosage between meals, over the course of the day, is most effective. A definitive study showed that a single low dose of phytosterols taken at the one morning meal was ineffective at lowering LDL cholesterol.[10] The study involved thirty subjects with high cholesterol, randomly assigned to consume one of four different types of phytosterol preparations, in a single dose at breakfast and compared to a control margarine with no added phytosterols. The phytosterol dosage ranged from 1.0 to 1.8 grams per day. After twenty-nine days, LDL cholesterol remained unchanged. The researchers hypothesized that because most cholesterol production by the liver occurs at night, blocking cholesterol absorption at the morning meal would not lead to optimal cholesterol reduction. Thus, this study reaffirms the importance of dividing the phytosterol daily dose between meals and taking a higher daily dose of phytosterols, at least 2 grams, for optimal cholesterol-lowering efficacy.

WHAT WORKS BETTER: STEROLS, STANOLS, OR BOTH TOGETHER?

Until more research clarifies which of the two types is more effective, sterols or stanols, or if they are equally effective, it would appear prudent to *aim for the NCEP goal of 2–3 grams per day of phytosterols.* To be on the safe side, I recommend that you try to mix up your sterols and stanols—most products and supplements contain a mixture of the two types, making consuming both easy to do. Just be sure to divide your phytosterol intake into two separate meals (with one meal being the evening one) and get in the minimum 2 grams per day.

PLANT STEROL CAVEATS

Count Your Calories

Don't think you can slather on the cholesterol-fighting margarine without paying the consequences on the scale! The regular margarines contain a whopping 90 calories per tablespoon. If you are not substituting the phytosterol-containing margarine for the fat you typically eat, over time you will gain weight from the added calories. The good news is that low-calorie phytosterol-containing products or supplements make it easy to get a daily dose of plant sterols without all the surplus calories. I recommend that you routinely eat the reduced-calorie phytosterol-containing margarines that weigh in at only 45 calories per tablespoon. Plus, they taste great! Three CholestOff Complete capsules contain a mere 20 calories.

Ten Tips for Adding Margarine with Phytosterols into Your Day

1. Butter your whole wheat bread with it.
2. Spread it on pancakes or waffles.
3. Fry your omelet (egg white, of course) or your grilled cheese (soy, of course) sandwich in it.
4. Butter your pasta (whole wheat, of course) with it.
5. Butter your corn on the cob with it.
6. Spruce up your steamed vegetables with it.
7. Add it to grain side dishes, such as brown rice or, better yet, barley.
8. Top your baked potato with it.
9. Sauté your garlic in it.
10. Melt it and pour it over your air-popped popcorn.

PHYTOSTEROLS SAFETY OVERVIEW

Phytosterols are on the FDA's list of substances that are generally recognized as safe (GRAS), meaning they have a long history of safe intake in humans without demonstrating harmful effects. GRAS clearance paved the way for commercial sales of phytosterol-containing products. To date, only two concerns have been addressed regarding the safety of phytosterol intake.

An extremely rare but serious genetic disorder exists in humans called sitosterolemia. People with this disorder have a defect in their intestinal cells that blocks excretion of the phytosterols back into the intestine, where they typically exit the body via the feces. Plant sterols/

stanols thus build up in the blood, causing premature atherosclerosis, often with fatal consequences. Obviously, people with sitosterolemia should not consume products with phytosterols.

Another concern regarding phytosterol intake is that it can reduce the absorption of fat-soluble vitamins A, E, D, and K and their precursors (carotenoids such as beta-carotene and alpha-carotene), because they are transported into the body in the same way as cholesterol. Researchers have suggested that to counteract this potential side effect, individuals should be vigilant about including lots of fruits and vegetables in their diet.[11] The National Cancer Institute, the National Institutes of Health, and the U.S. Department of Health and Human Services recommend five to nine servings of fruits and vegetables daily. Eating extra amounts of carotenoid- and lycopene-containing vegetables, such as carrots and tomatoes, is advised to offset the potential decrease in these nutrients with regular phytosterol intake.

FILLING THE PRESCRIPTION

Since the bulk of the scientific data have shown that the phytosterol-containing margarines are highly effective in reducing LDL cholesterol, I suggest that you try to include at least one serving of phytosterol-containing margarine on most days of the week. However, if the taste of margarine offends your palate or you don't want the extra calories found in the phytosterol-enriched margarines, then by all means take the supplements. CholestOff, manufactured by Nature Made, contains a blend of plant sterols and stanols. To obtain the recommended 2–3 grams per day, take the CholestOff Plus® Softgels, which require two capsules instead of three in the CholestOff Complete version. You need to consume six pills per day (I suggest taking three at lunch and three at dinner). It is available at drugstores as well as warehouse clubs such as Costco. Unfortunately, taking supplements will make a dent in your wallet as well as your cholesterol, but it may be worth it for the sake of convenience.

Once again, remember that the optimal dose recommended by NCEP for cholesterol-reduction benefits is 2–3 grams per day. Make sure to divide that up into two meals (one being the evening meal). Be aware that going over the upper goal range of 3 grams will *not* result in any further drop in cholesterol.

Functional Foods	Amount	Plant Sterols/Stanols
Promise Active Light Spread	1 tablespoon (45 calories)	1 gram plant sterol esters
Benecol Light Buttery Spreads	1 tablespoon (50 calories)	0.85 grams plant stanol esters
Benecol Smart Chews	4 chews (90 calories)	2 grams plant sterol esters

Supplement	Amount	Plant Sterols/Stanols
CholestOff Complete supplements	3 capsules	0.9 grams plant sterols and stanols
CholestOff Plus supplements	2 capsules	0.9 grams plant sterols and stanols

Phytosterols on the Internet

For more information on plant sterols and stanols or to order products online, log on to the following websites.

National Heart, Lung and Blood Institute (www.nhlbi.nih.gov)

American Heart Association (www.americanheart.org)

Food and Drug Administration (www.fda.gov)

Benecol (www.benecol.com)

Nature Made (www.naturemade.com)

CHAPTER 11

Step 8: Eat Soy Protein

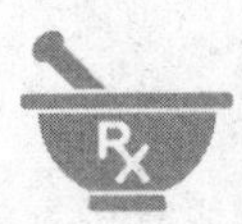

Eat 20–25 grams of soy protein every day.

"I don't like the taste of soy foods—is there any other way to get soy into my diet?" That's a typical response I get from patients when I recommend that they eat soy. "Keep an open mind," I tell them, as soy can be a delicious and beneficial addition to a healthful, varied diet. Unfortunately, many people don't realize that there is a whole world of tasty soy products on mainstream grocery shelves these days. It has become so much easier—and more palatable—to include these little legumes into our diets since tofu (soybean curd) first appeared in a U.S. supermarket in 1958. Forget vitamin pills—Americans who truly want to stay healthy and ward off disease should open their minds (and mouths) to the idea of adding soy to their daily diet.

WHY EAT SOY FOODS?

Not only do soybeans help protect against the number one killer of Americans, cardiovascular disease, but they have demonstrated tremendous potential in fighting off diseases on several other fronts. Frequent soy food consumption has been shown to:

- Lower cholesterol and thus reduce risk for heart disease and stroke
- Reduce risk for certain types of cancers such as breast, colon, and prostate
- Lower high blood pressure
- Preserve kidney function in diabetics as well as improve diabetes control
- Help keep bones healthy and prevent osteoporosis
- Potentially ease unpleasant symptoms of menopause
- Possibly prevent balding in men

The science supporting the connection between soy food consumption and heart health is so strong that the U.S. government recommends eating 25 grams of soy protein daily to help lower cholesterol. This federal recommendation stemmed from an analysis in 1995 of thirty-eight different studies, all concluding that soy protein consumption significantly lowers "bad" LDL cholesterol levels.[1] Since then, study after study has confirmed these findings. A recent meta-analysis[2] of forty-six controlled trials analyzing the effect of soy protein on LDL cholesterol found that consuming soy protein at a median dose of 25 grams per day significantly reduces LDL cholesterol by approximately 3–4 percent in adults.

Marla's Story

Marla G., age fifty-one
Pre: Total cholesterol: 284 mg/dL; LDL cholesterol: 211 mg/dL
Post: Total cholesterol: 201 mg/dL; LDL cholesterol: 140 mg/dL

34 percent reduction in LDL cholesterol

Marla is a personal trainer and marathon runner, but high cholesterol runs in her family. Although averse to taking any prescription medications, she reluctantly decided to try the lowest dose of a statin drug prescribed to treat her high

cholesterol. Almost immediately she began feeling nauseous and having severe muscle pains. She discontinued taking the medication. Here is what she had to say.

After discontinuing the statin drug, I was very concerned about my heart health, yet not knowing what else to try, I decided to attempt dieting one more time. I made an appointment with Dr. Brill and after several counseling sessions started on her Cholesterol Down Plan. At first I was resistant to the soy products; however, the other foods were appealing to me. Through trial and error, I found soy products that worked for me. It was easy to work in a daily Starbucks soy latte into my life.

Once I made a total commitment to changing my diet, it became easier and eventually just became a ritual part of my lifestyle. After four weeks following the plan, my "bad" cholesterol had dropped from 211 down to 140, 71 points. My doctor was absolutely amazed. I plan to continue eating this way for the rest of my life.

Like all beans, soybeans are highly nutritious, packed with all sorts of health-promoting ingredients. They are high in dietary fiber, B vitamins (including the heart-healthy folic acid), calcium, iron, phytochemicals (which protect against a host of diseases), and essential omega-3 fats. The composition of a soybean is 38 percent protein, 30 percent carbohydrate, 20 percent oil (mostly polyunsaturated), and the rest moisture. The protein found in soybeans is unique as plant sources of protein go: it's a high-quality protein, meaning it provides all the essential amino acids required in the human diet, and unlike animal protein, it contains zero cholesterol and only a minute amount of artery-clogging saturated fat.

NOT ALL SOY IS GOOD

You don't want to reach for the salad dressing made with soybean oil if you're looking to reap the phenomenal health benefits associated with soy foods. While Americans use massive quantities of soybean oil, a cheap source of fat that is ubiquitous in the world of processed foods, only soy foods in the form of soy protein confer substantial health benefits. You can avoid soybean oil (and in so doing lower your intake of the omega-6 fatty acid LA) by checking for it on food labels, but don't be misled, as soybean oil often is listed under the alias "vegetable oil."

How Much Does Soy Protein Really Lower LDL?

In an analysis of 22 studies by the American Heart Association, researchers found only an average 3 percent reduction in LDL cholesterol in participants who added soy protein to their diets. This casts some doubt on the more drastic reductions found by other studies, for instance, a large British study in which researchers at the University of Oxford examined the diets and blood work of more than 1,000 women participating in an arm of the European Prospective Investigation into Cancer and Nutrition Study. An average intake of 11 grams of soy protein per day was associated with a 12 percent lower LDL cholesterol level when compared to those women reporting an intake of less than 0.5 grams per day. Though the question remains as to exactly how much soy protein consumption lowers LDL, research seems to unanimously conclude that it does indeed lower it.

Source: Frank M. Sacks et al., "Soy Protein, Isoflavones, and Cardiovascular Health: An American Heart Association Science Advisory for Professionals from the Nutrition Committee," *Circulation* 113 (2006): 1034–1044; Magdalena S. Rosell et al., "Soy Intake and Blood Cholesterol Concentrations: A Cross-Sectional Study of 1033 Pre- and Postmenopausal Women in the Oxford Arm of the European Prospective Investigation into Cancer and Nutrition," *American Journal of Clinical Nutrition* 80 (2004): 1391–1396.

Soy sauce is also not the best choice for getting in your daily soy. Far from a healthful soy food product, soy sauce contains an enormous amount of sodium, yet only a minimal amount of health-promoting, active soy ingredients.

WHAT EXACTLY IS IN SOYBEANS THAT LOWERS CHOLESTEROL?

The heart-healthy benefits of soy are well documented and are attributed to several actions involving phytoestrogens, antioxidants, and amino acids. Here is a synopsis of the mechanisms tied to the cholesterol-lowering effects of soy.

Method of Attack #1. A meta-analysis of eight studies concluded that the component of soy protein most responsible for lowering cholesterol is the phytoestrogens.[3] Phytoestrogens (soy-derived phytoestrogens are known as isoflavones) are plant-derived chemicals that are structurally very similar to the female hormone estrogen and can therefore exert weak hormone-like effects in the body. Estrogen is known to protect premenopausal women from heart disease, and the phytoestrogens work in much the same way—by increasing the number and effectiveness of LDL cholesterol receptors on the liver, in turn increasing their ability to take up and dispose of cholesterol from the bloodstream.[4]

Method of Attack #2. The strong antioxidant capability of phytoestrogens helps soy reduce the risk of heart attack and stroke. LDL cholesterol circulating in the bloodstream is relatively harmless unless it settles within the arterial wall and becomes oxidized, contributing to inflammation, plaque buildup, and ultimately a heart attack. Arteries damaged by plaque buildup have a narrowing of the pathway for blood flow. If a blood clot develops, it essentially seals off the flow of blood. In an artery leading to the heart muscle, this can lead to a heart attack. If the process occurs in arteries serving the brain, the result is a stroke. Soy's antioxidant properties make this legume an ally in the fight against oxidation of LDL cholesterol and the prevention of plaque buildup.

Method of Attack #3. Soy protein has been shown to have a beneficial effect on the size and shape of the LDL cholesterol particles. Small and dense LDL particles are associated with a much greater risk of heart disease than larger particles, because they can easily pass into the inner layer of the arteries via minute cracks between cells. This inner layer is where LDL particles contribute to the plaque formation that is the hallmark of atherosclerosis. According to new research, soy protein consumption increases the size of LDL particles so that fewer of them enter the arterial inner layer, hence a less risky form of circulating "bad" cholesterol.[5]

Method of Attack #4. Soy protein's amino acid profile also contributes to its cholesterol-lowering and cardioprotective properties. The FDA states that the amino acid content of soy "is different from animal protein and most other vegetable proteins and appears to alter the synthesis and metabolism of cholesterol in the liver."[6] Soy protein is rich in the amino acid arginine, which is healthful for the arteries. It is a precursor to nitric oxide, the substance that helps to dilate arteries and increase their flexibility, thereby decreasing the potential for a heart attack by a blood clot. Some scientists believe soy's arginine content explains the link between soy and substantial heart health benefits. Researchers out of the University of Milan, Italy, suggest that it may have been the high arginine-to-lysine ratio in soy protein that was responsible for the dramatic cholesterol-clearing results of their study. Twelve individuals with high cholesterol were placed on a standard low-fat diet with added animal protein for four weeks, then switched to the same[7] low-fat diet but this time with soy protein in place of the animal protein, for four weeks. Following the soy protein diet, LDL was lowered by 16 percent compared to no change following the animal protein diet. What's more, the soy protein diet significantly increased the number and effectiveness of LDL receptors.

Method of Attack #5. Soy contains a large protein (proteins consist of long strings of amino acids all linked together) called 7S globulin. Scientists surmise that once ingested, the protein is broken down in the intestine into smaller strands of amino acids that escape further digestion, entering the bloodstream intact. Research suggests that these special enzyme-resistant soy protein by-products interfere with LDL metabolism (activating liver LDL receptors), the end result being a decline in blood LDL cholesterol.[8] Furthermore, a team of Italian researchers showed that 7S globulin also affects beta-VLDL liver receptors, leading to increased clearance of these final-stage LDL precursor compounds.[9]

Method of Attack #6. By adding soy protein to your diet, you tend to eliminate some animal protein, which is loaded with saturated fat and cholesterol. Cut your saturated fat and cholesterol intake and you automatically lower LDL cholesterol. A diet high in animal protein can actually induce high LDL cholesterol, at least according to animal research. Rabbits fed an animal protein chow (high in the milk protein casein) showed a higher rate of production of Apo B protein (the type that encircles LDL particles) and LDL cholesterol compared with rabbits fed chow high in soy protein.[10]

SOY CAUTION

Disadvantages of eating soy foods appear to affect only individuals with known food allergies or individuals diagnosed with some type of thyroid dysfunction. Soy does tend to be a highly allergenic food, particularly in children, so if you're sensitive to soy, avoid eating soy products. Soy may also cause problems with thyroid function by deactivating the enzyme responsible for synthesizing thyroid hormones. Some scientific evidence even suggests a link between soy consumption and goiter, but the consensus is that in healthy individuals, soy consumption does not adversely affect thyroid function. If you've been diagnosed with thyroid dysfunction, exert caution in consuming soy products.

Soy foods can also be high in fat and calories. A cup of full-fat soy milk contains 127 calories and 5 grams of fat. That's 40 more calories and 5 more grams of fat than a glass of fat-free milk. Soy nuts are a tasty way to add soy into your day but, like all nuts, are high in calories;

eat too many and you'll pay at the scale. Soy cereals taste great—but beware, they are often sugar-coated.

Breast Cancer Survivors Are Encouraged to Eat Soy

Major cancer organizations, including the American Cancer Society and the American Institute for Cancer Research, endorse soy consumption for breast cancer survivors. Current research reveals no evidence linking soy foods to increased recurrence risk or adverse outcomes in survivors. Emerging studies actually point toward potential benefits—particularly from isoflavone-rich soy products—suggesting these foods may lower recurrence rates and contribute to improved long-term survival outcomes.

A groundbreaking 2024 meta-analysis from the Johns Hopkins Kimmel Cancer Center revealed striking survival benefits for breast cancer survivors who consume soy foods. Published in January 2024 in JNCI Cancer Spectrum, the comprehensive review analyzed twenty-two observational studies and found that soy isoflavones were associated with a 26 percent reduction in the risk of breast cancer recurrence among 11,837 women across six studies. The protective effects proved most pronounced in postmenopausal survivors and reached optimal benefit levels at specific dosages. The greatest risk reduction was seen at 60 mg per day, equivalent to two to three servings per day, where one serving equates to a cup of soy milk, three ounces of tofu, or a half-cup of cooked soybeans.

Source: M. Diana van Die et al., "Phytonutrients and Outcomes Following Breast Cancer: A Systematic Review and Meta-Analysis of Observational Studies," *JNCI Cancer Spectrum* 8, no. 1 (2024), https://doi.org/10.1093/jncics/pkad104.

FILLING THE PRESCRIPTION

Americans should include soy foods in their diet on a daily basis, to the tune of *20–25 grams of soy protein per day.* My patients find it easiest to simply replace cow's milk with soy milk. Another tasty option is edamame (pronounced ay-duh-MAH-may), which you can order at Japanese restaurants or purchase frozen at your local health food store or grocery store and cook at home in your microwave.

Many patients even enjoy dropping by Starbucks and ordering a soy latte to help fill their daily soy prescription. A "tall" latte provides 11 ounces of Silk soy milk, or approximately 9 grams of soy protein; a "grande" provides approximately 12 grams of soy protein and a "venti" approximately 15 grams, respectively. Getting 20–25 grams of soy protein into your day is easy; you can do the math and put together a daily combination of foods that will make a large impact on your cholesterol-lowering regimen.

Soy Food	Amount	Soy Protein
Tempeh	½ cup (4 ounces) (200 calories)	19 grams
Tofu (firm)	½ cup (4 ounces) (70 calories)	13–20 grams
Edamame or "sweet beans"	½ cup (40 calories)	11 grams
Soy nuts (dry-roasted)	¼ cup (250 calories)	10–15 grams
Soy crumbles	½ cup (55 calories)	9 grams
Soy nut butter	2 tablespoons (170 calories)	8 grams
Plain soy milk	8 ounces (125 calories)	7–10 grams
Soy flour	¼ cup (90 calories)	7 grams
Soy "burger"	1 (125 calories)	4–10 grams
Soy "sausage"	2 links (80 calories)	2–6 grams

Soy on the Internet

For more information, delicious recipes, and to find out just about anything else you would like to know about soy, I suggest the following information sources on the Web.

United Soybean Board (www.unitedsoybean.org)

Indiana Soybean Alliance (https://soybeanresearchinfo.com/states/indiana)

U.S. Soyfoods Directory (www.soyfoods.com)

Silk (www.silk.com)

Boca Foods (www.kraftheinz.com/boca/products/00759283334455-original-vegan-veggie-burgers)

Morningstar Farms (www.morningstarfarms.com/en_US/home.html)

CHAPTER 12

Step 9: Eat Fewer Calories

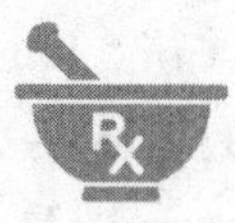

Cut typical daily calorie intake by 10 percent.

Of all the steps in the Cholesterol Down Plan, eating fewer calories—or practicing calorie restriction—is perhaps the most powerful and makes the most dramatic dent in your LDL cholesterol level. Yet for many it is the most difficult step. Let's face it, in our food-centric world, eating fewer calories is hard to do.

Calorie restriction is defined as a sustained dietary regimen (typically lasting six months or longer) that involves lowering your average daily caloric intake below what is typical for you, without depriving yourself of essential nutrients or becoming malnourished. Unlike temporary dieting approaches focused on short-term weight loss goals, calorie restriction represents a permanent lifestyle adjustment—a way of eating that you maintain indefinitely rather than something you stop once you reach a target weight.

In humans, calorie restriction usually involves reducing your caloric intake by 10 percent or more from what you typically eat and maintaining this lower calorie intake for an extended period. Calorie restriction is a wide-open field of study, with many scientists suggesting that following this dietary regime can help you ward off aging and diseases and extend your life.

Again, keep in mind that calorie restriction regimens are not temporary weight-loss plans, nor are they starvation diets. While healthful calorie restriction programs can help you maintain or reach a healthy body weight, the scale alone doesn't tell the whole story of your health improvements. The primary goal of calorie restriction isn't necessarily weight loss per se but rather reducing harmful visceral fat—the dangerous abdominal fat that surrounds your organs and drives inflammation—while preserving lean muscle mass.

Whether you're currently overweight or at a healthy weight, calorie restriction offers significant cardiovascular benefits by reducing visceral fat, lowering inflammation, and improving metabolic function. For those at normal weight, research shows that modest calorie restriction—typically 10–15 percent below maintenance needs—can lower LDL cholesterol and improve heart disease risk factors even without significant weight loss. While some initial weight loss may occur, many normal-weight individuals find their weight stabilizes at a slightly lower but still healthy level while continuing to reap the metabolic benefits. This chapter explores how moderate, sustainable calorie reduction can benefit virtually anyone seeking to optimize their heart health—with the important exceptions of those who are underweight or children, for whom calorie restriction would not be appropriate.

Sam's Story

Samuel D., age fifty-three
Pre: Total cholesterol: 162 mg/dL; LDL cholesterol: 101 mg/dL
Post: Total cholesterol: 128 mg/dL; LDL cholesterol: 62 mg/dL

39 percent reduction in LDL cholesterol

Sam is a middle-aged professional with a type A personality and a strong family history of heart disease. His father had a heart attack before the age of fifty, and his grandfather died of the disease in his thirties. Concerned about his heart health, he had a preventive angiogram several years ago. Despite receiving a clean bill of health, he suffered a heart attack at age fifty-one. His doctor placed him on a statin medication, but he

was not having much success getting his LDL down to under 70 mg/dL and whittling away his dangerous belly fat. Here is what Sam had to say.

The irony wasn't lost on me. I'd done everything right—maintained a healthy diet, exercised when I could, never touched a cigarette. The preventive angiogram gave me false confidence. When the heart attack hit, it felt like a betrayal by my own body.

The stent saved my life, and taking the statin became my new reality. But I knew I needed more. My doctor wanted my LDL below 70 mg/dL, yet even with medication, those numbers remained stubbornly high. The belly fat I'd accumulated over the years seemed equally resistant to change.

That's when I discovered Dr. Brill's Cholesterol Down Plan. My doctor also suggested I combine the heart-healthy lifestyle plan with a GLP-1 medication—thankfully covered by my insurance. This combination transformed everything. Wegovy didn't just suppress my appetite; it rewired my relationship with food. Suddenly, choosing nutritious options felt natural rather than forced. The Cholesterol Down Plan seamlessly integrated into this new lifestyle.

My routine became sustainable: thirty minutes of daily walking, twice-weekly weight training, and yoga for the stress that had always been my companion. Within four weeks, the transformation was undeniable—twelve pounds of fat gone, my waistline visibly reduced, and that stunning 39 percent drop in LDL cholesterol.

The numbers tell the story, but the feeling tells it better. For the first time since my heart attack, I feel like I'm winning the fight my genes started.

CALORIE RESTRICTION AND HEART HEALTH

Calorie restriction is a powerful means to lower your LDL cholesterol and promote healthy aging, even in individuals not considered overweight. But how exactly does eating less affect your body?

Scientists are collecting some interesting data that could offer the long-sought-after answer. The following is an overview of the different hypothesized mechanisms related to the ability of calorie restriction to benefit your health.

FROM MICE TO MEN (AND WOMEN): THE CALERIE STUDY

You may have heard of the phenomenal health effects of cutting calorie intake in mice and how it is a proven intervention to slow down the aging process. What you may not know is that a randomized clinical trial (the strongest type of research study) exposing humans to a long-term program of calorie restriction has recently produced evidence of improved disease resistance.

The CALERIE™ study[1] (CALERIE is an acronym for "Comprehensive Assessment of Long-Term Effects of Reducing Intake of Energy") is the first-ever study to focus specifically on the effects of sustained calorie restriction in healthy adults ages 21–50 years. Funded by the U.S. National Institute on Aging, the study randomly assigned 220 men and women at three sites in the U.S. to a 25 percent calorie-restriction or normal diet for two years. Results showed subjects achieved two years of an approximately 12 percent calorie restriction from baseline.

The results? Nothing short of remarkable—the calorie restriction group lost an average of 17 pounds and significantly reduced LDL cholesterol by approximately 11 mg/dL. But the benefits extended far beyond cholesterol numbers. Those who reduced their caloric intake also experienced meaningful reductions in waist circumference, which is particularly important since belly fat is strongly linked to heart disease risk. Their blood pressure dropped to healthier levels, and many saw improvements in other cardiovascular markers like triglycerides and HDL (good) cholesterol ratios. Furthermore, calorie restriction resulted in a significant decrease in inflammatory markers in the bloodstream, which may be the mechanism responsible for slowing age-related decline and improving disease resistance.

What makes these findings especially compelling is that participants weren't following extreme diets—they were simply eating fewer of their regular foods while maintaining good nutrition. The study demonstrated that calorie restriction works like a master key, unlocking multiple pathways to better heart health simultaneously. Rather than targeting just one risk factor, reducing calories creates a cascade of positive changes throughout the cardiovascular system.

This research provides strong scientific backing for the idea that "eating less" can be just as powerful as complex medical interventions when it comes to protecting your heart. The beauty lies in its simplicity—by consuming fewer calories while maintaining nutritional quality, people can address multiple cardiovascular risk factors with a single lifestyle change. The study authors note that calorie restriction, started at young and middle age, may prolong your staying healthy longer by delaying disease development and even extend your life.

It is important to note that the CALERIE study included some normal-weight participants, and they experienced cardiovascular benefits such as improved cholesterol, blood pressure, and inflammatory markers as well. However, the approach requires careful monitoring for normal-weight individuals, and the focus should be on nutrient density—getting maximum nutrition from fewer calories rather than simply eating less food. Also, when people practice long-term calorie restriction, they don't continue losing weight indefinitely—instead, their body reaches a new equilibrium through a process called metabolic adaptation. Initially, reducing calories by 10–15 percent will cause some weight loss (even in normal-weight individuals), but over 6 to 12 months, the metabolism gradually adjusts downward to match the reduced caloric intake. The CALERIE study demonstrated this exact pattern: participants lost weight during the first six months but then stabilized at a lower weight without continuing to shed pounds. What was once a calorie deficit becomes the new maintenance level—for example, someone previously maintaining weight at 2,000 calories might find that 1,700 calories becomes their new normal after metabolic adaptation. This protective mechanism prevents people from wasting away on long-term restriction. The body essentially becomes more metabolically efficient, allowing people to maintain their health improvements without the concern of endless weight loss.

EXCESS BODY FAT AND LDL LEVELS

If you are overweight—defined as having excess body fat—you are more likely to have elevated LDL and to develop diabetes and heart disease. Individuals who store fat around the midsection are at the greatest risk for these diseases. If you are overweight, losing just 5 to 10 percent of your current body weight is one of the most powerful actions you can take to dramatically lower your LDL cholesterol. Weight loss of about 20 pounds has been shown to reduce LDL by a whopping 15 percent. If you are overweight, this step in the Cholesterol Down Plan will surely be one of the most valuable additions to your LDL-lowering arsenal.

Sadly, if you struggle with being overweight, you are not alone. The fact is that the vast majority, some 74 percent of adult Americans, are classified as overweight. This is a major problem for our heart health. Why? Because extra body fat raises your chances of having too much LDL floating in your bloodstream. Every 10 pounds of extra weight (in the form of body fat, not muscle) causes your body to produce as much as 10 mg of extra cholesterol every single day. Overweight (excess body fat) causes chronic inflammation that contributes to the process of atherosclerosis (plaque buildup) and premature death.[2]

Where you store body fat also affects your cholesterol level and risk of disease. The extra pounds that tend to park themselves around the midsection are the most dangerous, so as our waistlines grow, so do our health risks. There are two kinds of body fat: subcutaneous fat and visceral fat. Subcutaneous fat (the less dangerous type) is the fat found directly beneath the skin throughout the body, forming a layer between the skin and the underlying muscle. It's the fat you can pinch or grab with your fingers. The fat inside your belly (the visceral fat) can be seen and measured but not pinched. Visceral fat (also called belly fat or abdominal fat) lies out of reach, deep within the abdominal cavity, where it pads the spaces between our abdominal organs. It is of particular concern. If you store fat around your abdomen rather than your hips and thighs, you have a significantly increased risk for developing heart disease and type 2 diabetes. This risk goes up with a waist size that is greater than 35 inches for women or greater than 40 inches for men. Refer to the end of this chapter for online site instructions to accurately measure your waist circumference.

DEFINING OVERWEIGHT

Scientists have traditionally screened for weight categories that may lead to health problems using the body mass index (BMI). Your BMI is a number calculated from your weight and your height. While BMI is an imperfect clinical measure when it comes to assessing body fat, it is a quick, inexpensive, and easy-to-calculate tool to get a general idea of whether someone might be classified as underweight, overweight, or obese. (You can easily calculate your BMI yourself by inserting your height and weight into the National Heart, Lung, and Blood Institute online BMI calculator listed at the end of this chapter.) A healthy body weight is categorized as having a BMI between 18.5 and 25. A BMI *above 25* is considered overweight and strongly predisposes you to having elevated LDL cholesterol.

That said, BMI has come under fire lately, as it has flaws. BMI does not consider muscle mass, bone density, overall body composition, or racial and gender differences, nor does it account for the fact that muscle weighs more than fat. BMI is associated with but is not a direct measure of body fat and does not assess health risks related to body fat distribution.

A replacement metric called the body roundness index or BRI has been gaining support. The BRI is a better measure of abdominal fat, which is more closely linked to disease. New science backs this notion up. A recent study[3] published in *JAMA Network Open* shows it to be more accurate than BMI for predicting health risk. The BRI is a measure of how round or circle-like you are, using a formula that takes into account weight, height, *and* hip and waist circumference. To calculate your BRI, plug your weight, height, and waist and hip circumference into the online BRI calculator listed at the end of this chapter. A healthy BRI typically falls between 1 and 16. Lower BRI values, closer to 1, indicate less body fat and a healthier body composition, whereas higher values suggest more visceral fat and a greater chance of health issues.

Sources: Centers for Disease Control and Prevention, "About Body Mass Index (BMI)," July 17, 2024, www.cdc.gov/bmi/about/index.html; Xiaoqian Zhang et al., "Body Roundness Index and All-Cause Mortality Among US Adults," *JAMA Network Open* 7, no. 6 (June 5, 2024): e2415051, https://doi.org/10.1001/jamanetworkopen.2024.15051.

HOW DOES CALORIE RESTRICTION LOWER LDL CHOLESTEROL?

Calorie restriction has emerged as one of the most effective dietary strategies for improving cholesterol levels and overall cardiovascular health. Research consistently shows that reducing caloric intake, even modestly, can lead to significant improvements in cholesterol profiles, particularly in lowering harmful LDL cholesterol levels. Restricting calories lowers LDL cholesterol through several powerful mechanisms.

Method of Attack #1. Calorie restriction lowers your cholesterol levels because it can reduce the amount of fat you have in your body. Body fat is the main determinant of metabolic abnormalities and produces a chronic inflammatory state that promotes heart disease. Total body fat is the best predictor of C-reactive protein levels[4] (a blood marker of inflammation). Reduce the amount of body fat, and you quell the inflammation.

Method of Attack #2. Oxidative stress is the term used to describe what occurs when the body has too many volatile molecules called free radicals and not enough antioxidants to neutralize them. This chronic imbalance can lead to cell damage, premature aging, disease, and a shortened lifespan. Oxidation of LDL is the first step in the cascade of events leading to plaque formation. Calorie restriction fights off this oxidative stress as well as decrease inflammation, two key factors in the process of atherosclerosis, by reducing the production of free radicals in cell walls and strengthening the cells against oxidative damage. Calorie restriction has also been shown to enhance the body's antioxidant systems, including increasing vitamin E regeneration and improving how our body uses vitamin C to support antioxidant processes.[5]

Method of Attack #3. Losing weight (especially body fat) and being more active reverses insulin resistance so your body is better able to regulate hormones and lipoproteins. Excess body fat, especially around the abdomen, is a major cause of insulin resistance. Insulin resistance (primarily seen in liver and skeletal muscle cells) is caused by excessive fat accumulation in those cells. Muscle insulin resistance leads to increased blood triglycerides and LDL, which are major contributors to heart disease. The development of insulin resistance also marks the beginning of diabetes. By practicing a long-term calorie restriction program, you can reverse insulin resistance, making the muscle cells more sensitive to blood sugar, and open the door for blood sugar transport into the muscle cell. Losing body fat from calorie restriction can normalize the storage of ingested carbohydrate into the muscle as glycogen, decreasing the conversion of carbohydrate to fat in the liver. This, in turn, leads to a decrease in the liver's production of LDL cholesterol, which will protect against the development of atherosclerosis. According to research,[6] losing approximately 7 percent of your excess body weight can significantly reduce the risk of developing type 2 diabetes by close to 60 percent!

CALORIE RESTRICTION CAUTION

Unfortunately, several forms of calorie restriction can carry potential risks. First, people with eating disorders are vulnerable to excessive and dangerous weight loss. Second, consuming fewer calories increases the risk of inadequate intake of nutrients. Third, rapid weight loss from consuming too few calories may lead to loss of muscle and bone tissue, which can cause unfavorable changes in physical functionality. The following groups of people should not practice any method of calorie restriction: underweight people or people with eating disorders; those who are pregnant, trying to conceive, and breastfeeding; children; and older adults with gait issues. The following groups of people can practice calorie restriction but only under medical supervision: those with type 1 or 2 diabetes, those taking prescription medications, or those with diagnosed underlying medical conditions.

Normal-weight individuals considering calorie restriction should proceed with significant caution and medical supervision. While modest calorie reduction (10–15 percent below your current maintenance level) may offer metabolic benefits, normal-weight people face heightened risks of nutrient deficiencies, muscle loss, and hormonal disruption since they lack excess fat stores to buffer nutritional gaps. Essential safeguards for all individuals choosing to practice long-term calorie restriction include prioritizing nutrient-dense foods, ensuring adequate protein intake to preserve lean muscle mass, maintaining resistance exercise, and obtaining regular medical monitoring of nutritional status, bone density, and metabolic markers. For normal-weight individuals, the focus should remain on achieving metabolic health improvements rather than further weight loss, with careful attention to preventing the development of obsessive food behaviors or nutritional deficiencies that could outweigh any potential benefits.

FILLING THE PRESCRIPTION

If you are overweight, you need to reduce body fat and lose weight for better health. What is the best way to achieve this? Scientists have confirmed repeatedly that eating a healthy reduced-calorie diet and combining that with a daily exercise regimen will help you attain the recommended amount of weight loss: 5 to 10 percent of your current body weight. A healthy and sustainable rate of weight loss is generally around 0.5 to 1 percent of your body weight per week, a rate that focuses on losing primarily body fat rather than muscle mass. However, the principles of calorie management and metabolic health discussed in this section apply to everyone—including normal-weight individuals who may benefit from understanding how calorie restriction can improve cardiovascular health, enhance cellular repair processes, and optimize metabolic function without the goal of weight loss. Whether your goal is fat loss or metabolic optimization, you need to manage your caloric intake strategically and maintain consistent physical activity. Despite what you may have heard, calories do count for everyone.

For sustainable weight loss, slow and steady wins the race. When you lose weight at a rate of only one to two pounds a week—you lose almost exclusively body fat. (Healthy weight loss targets loss of fat, not muscle.) Preserving muscle mass is important, as muscle tissue burns significantly more calories at rest than fat tissue, so preserving muscle during weight loss helps maintain your metabolic rate and prevents weight regain. Additionally, muscle mass is essential for maintaining bone health. Furthermore, age-related muscle loss (sarcopenia) progressively reduces quality of life by limiting mobility, increasing fall risk, and making everyday activities like climbing stairs, carrying groceries, or getting up from chairs increasingly difficult. This muscle deterioration also contributes to frailty, loss of independence, and higher rates of hospitalization and disability in older adults.

Creating a sustainable calorie deficit of approximately 500 calories per day has traditionally been recommended for losing one pound of body fat per week. To accomplish a daily 500-calorie deficit, you can try eating 250 calories less than you normally eat and then burning an additional 250 calories with exercise (refer to Chapter 13 to see how easy it is to burn 250 calories with walking). I have also included a website at the end of this chapter that calculates the approximate number of calories burned when you walk for exercise using your body weight and a walking speed calculator. This is a sensible weight loss regimen—diet fads come and go, but sensible weight loss techniques stand the test of time. However, research shows that even smaller deficits of 300–400 calories daily can provide significant health benefits, including improved cardiovascular markers and metabolic function. This holds true for all adults, whether their goal is weight loss or optimizing health at their current weight.

INTERMITTENT FASTING: AN EFFECTIVE WAY TO CUT CALORIES

Many, if not most of us, find it extremely difficult to adhere to a low-calorie diet over the long term. Enter intermittent fasting. Over the past decade, intermittent fasting has emerged as a promising alternative to low-calorie diets that promote increased compliance and improvements in heart health parameters.

Yes, intermittent fasting can facilitate eating less and losing weight and, in so doing, reducing LDL. Intermittent fasting is currently one of the most popular health and fitness trends in the world. It is not a diet but an eating schedule. Intermittent fasting plans tell you when to eat rather than what to eat. There are many ways to practice intermittent fasting, with the 16:8 method being the simplest version (eating is confined to an 8-hour window with 16 hours of fasting, every day). If you are new to intermittent fasting, I suggest you begin with this method.

Regardless of how long your window for eating is, intermittent fasting is effective for weight loss. A Canadian meta-analysis[7] (a statistical method for combining data from multiple studies to reach a single conclusion) examined twenty-seven scientific studies involving intermittent fasting and weight loss in overweight people. Results showed that all forms of intermittent fasting resulted in weight loss, ranging from 1 percent to 13 percent of baseline body weight.

It is a more sustainable method for reducing calorie intake. Many people vastly prefer to have periods of unrestricted food intake to be interwoven with differing periods of fasting than follow traditional diets. As a result, we see more longer-term compliance with intermittent fasting.

Not overweight? Intermittent fasting can still reduce LDL. If you have elevated LDL but do not need to lose weight, an Australian study[8] has shown that the process of intermittent fasting itself targets LDL cholesterol independent of weight loss. Researchers compared two groups of overweight people following either a regular reduced-calorie diet or a program of intermittent fasting for 12 weeks. Results showed that the reductions in total and LDL cholesterol were greater in the intermittent fasting group without statistically significant weight loss. The likely explanation is that intermittent fasting triggers beneficial changes in how the liver processes fats and cholesterol—essentially "resetting" the body's fat-burning machinery to work more efficiently, which improves cholesterol levels independently of weight loss.

The Steadfast Laws of Physics and Weight Loss

Newton's First Law of Thermodynamics is the law of conservation of energy. This law states that in a closed system, energy cannot be created or destroyed. Translation: If the calories in the foods you eat exceed the number of calories your body burns and you do this consistently, you create what is called a calorie surplus. Over time, you will gain weight (fat). If you eat fewer calories from food than your body expends on a consistent basis, you create a calorie deficit, and you will lose weight. All diets (low-carb, low-fat, Mediterranean, Paleo, plant-based, etc.) work by creating a sustained calorie deficit—regardless of how many carbs, fats, and proteins you eat. If you don't create a sustained calorie deficit, you will not lose weight. If you create too great a calorie deficit, you lose both muscle mass and body fat, which is not the desired weight loss composition. It's a balancing act: you need to create a deficit without going overboard.

In recent years, some diet advocates have claimed that calories don't matter—that hormones, food timing, or specific macronutrients are what really determine weight loss. Social media is rife with influencers promoting the idea that you can eat unlimited amounts of certain "good" foods and still lose weight or that counting calories is outdated. Debating the fundamental role of energy balance in weight regulation—and the "calories in, calories out" approach to weight management—is an exercise in futility, an argument with Sir Isaac Newton. No one can defy the first law of thermodynamics. That said, it is true that the number of calories required to lose weight or to maintain a weight loss or gain differs from person to person, influenced by numerous factors beyond our control such as genetics, socioeconomic status, environmental factors, and mental health. These factors contribute to the complex web of weight loss challenges that affect us.

Sources: Kevin D. Hall, "Thermodynamics of Weight Loss Diets," *Nutrition and Metabolism* 1, no. 1 (December 2004): 15, https://doi.org/10.1186/1743-7075-1-15; David Albuquerque et al., "The Contribution of Genetics and Environment to Obesity," *British Medical Bulletin* 123, no. 1 (September 2017): 159–173, https://doi.org/10.1093/bmb/ldx022.

CALORIE COUNTING: A TIME-TESTED METHOD FOR CALORIE RESTRICTION

Calorie counting can be particularly valuable for achieving calorie restriction because it provides precision and accountability that many people need to create and maintain the necessary calorie deficit. When trying to reduce calorie intake, calorie counting helps ensure you're actually in a deficit rather than just estimating, which is crucial since many people underestimate their intake by 20–40 percent. It serves as an educational tool that teaches you what portion sizes look like, reveals hidden calories in foods and beverages, and helps identify eating patterns that may be sabotaging progress.

Additionally, calorie counting provides objective data that allows for systematic adjustments—if your LDL cholesterol isn't improving as expected, you can make informed modifications to your intake rather than guessing. The method works particularly well for detail-oriented individuals who find numbers motivating rather than stressful, those who benefit from structure and concrete data, and people who prefer flexibility in food choices within a defined calorie budget.

If you're very physically active, keeping tabs on calorie intake will ensure you're consuming adequate energy for performance and recovery. Even loose monitoring can help verify that you're eating at maintenance levels rather than creating an unintended deficit that could lead to a large unwanted weight loss. If you notice significant changes in weight, energy levels, or overall well-being, some basic tracking can help you adjust portion sizes appropriately. The key is ensuring you meet your nutritional needs while still gaining the metabolic benefits of calorie restriction.

However, this approach is not recommended for those with a history of obsessive food behaviors where counting could trigger unhealthy patterns; children and adolescents; and people who practice mindful eating and respond well to hunger and satiety cues. For these individuals, the potential risks of calorie counting—including increased food anxiety, obsessive behaviors, or emotional distress—outweigh the benefits. Those with a history of disordered eating should be especially cautious, as calorie counting can reactivate harmful patterns even years after recovery.

Ideally, calorie counting should serve as a temporary educational tool rather than a permanent lifestyle requirement, with the goal of developing sustainable eating patterns and portion awareness that eventually allow for intuitive, healthy choices without constant monitoring. Think of it as training wheels—helpful for learning but not meant to be permanent. It is critical to ensure that you're still meeting all your nutritional requirements when reducing calories.

For intermittent fasting aimed at health benefits rather than weight loss, detailed calorie calculations are typically unnecessary as well. The time restriction method itself often naturally regulates intake, and your primary focus should be on the metabolic benefits like improved insulin sensitivity and cellular repair rather than precise calorie counting. This approach works particularly well for simple schedules like 16:8, where you eat normally during your designated eating window.

DOING THE CALORIE CALCULATIONS (IF IT'S RIGHT FOR YOU)

If you'd like to use calorie counting, your first step is to calculate the number of calories you need to eat (and the number of calories you burn based on your activity level) to maintain your current body weight. Once you have that number, you calculate what your daily intake would be if you reduce it by 10 percent, which you can do by multiplying this number by 0.9. The result is the number of calories you should eat to maintain a long-term plan of calorie restriction.

For example, if your body requires 2,000 calories to maintain your current body weight, you will need to reduce your calorie intake to 1,800 calories a day (while maintaining your current activity level) as a guideline for your healthy calorie restriction plan. Thankfully, the American Cancer Society has an online calorie counter tool that makes doing the calculations simple. Refer to the end of this chapter for access to this and other helpful calorie restriction sites.

Remember that calorie counting is just one method among several for achieving calorie restriction. Whether it becomes a helpful tool or a source of stress depends largely on your individual personality, history with food, and current relationship with eating. The best approach is always the one you can maintain over the long term without compromising your physical or emotional well-being.

WEIGHT LOSS DRUGS: WHAT YOU NEED TO KNOW

In recent years, GLP-1 receptor agonists have exploded in popularity despite their prohibitive cost. It's no surprise—these drugs make the incredibly arduous task of eating fewer calories easier. New research shows that the ability of these drugs to enable people to restrict calories over the long term translates into major weight loss and a significant reduction in LDL cholesterol. A Hungarian study published in the prestigious journal *Atherosclerosis* proves this point. Eleven people received 1 mg of semaglutide (Ozempic) per week for the six-month research period. The result? A significant reduction in body weight occurred in all participants in addition to a dramatic decline in the amount of small, dense LDL cholesterol (the most dangerous type).

FIRST, WHAT ARE THESE DRUGS?

There are many medications on the market that fall under the umbrella of GLP-1 receptor agonists. GLP-1 agonists are not new, and they were initially developed to treat type 2 diabetes. When clinical trials showed that diabetes patients taking GLP-1 agonists were losing substantial amounts of weight due to their appetite-suppressing effects, pharmaceutical companies began developing higher-dose formulations specifically for obesity treatment.

GLP-1 stands for glucagon-like peptide 1, a hormone produced in the intestinal system and released when you eat food. GLP-1 works by telling your brain that you have eaten enough food. Normally, this signal comes and goes in minutes. What the medications do is mimic the effects of GLP-1 but make the signal last for far longer time periods, helping you feel full and decreasing appetite. They also slow down food passing through the digestive tract, adding to the feeling of fullness. People on these drugs lose weight quickly because they consume fewer calories.

These medications are a game changer in the field of weight management. They work on the brain, mimicking essential gut hormones that control eating behavior, nutritional absorption, digestion, and the overall balance of calories coming into and being used by the body. While discontinuing these medications can lead to weight regain, successful long-term outcomes depend on using the treatment period to establish sustainable eating habits, appropriate portion sizes, and regular physical activity—the same lifestyle foundations that support lasting weight management regardless of medication use.

Weight Loss in a Syringe

Here is a list of GLP-1 receptor agonist medications currently on the U.S. market:

- Exenatide (brand names Byetta and Bydureon, manufactured by AstraZeneca)
- Liraglutide (Victoza for diabetes, Saxenda for obesity, manufactured by Novo Nordisk)
- Albiglutide (Tanzeum, manufactured by GSK)
- Dulaglutide (Trulicity, manufactured by Eli Lilly)
- Lixisenatide (Lyxumia in Europe, Adlyxin in the United States, manufactured by Sanofi)
- Semaglutide (Ozempic and Rybelsus for diabetes, Wegovy for obesity, manufactured by Novo Nordisk)
- Tirzepatide (dual GLP-1 and GIP agonist; Mounjaro for diabetes, Zepbound for obesity, manufactured by Eli Lilly)

Note: Most of these medications are administered as weekly subcutaneous injections, though Rybelsus (oral semaglutide) is already available as a daily pill for diabetes. Clinical trials for oral versions of other GLP-1 medications are showing promising results, suggesting that more pill options may become available in the near future for those who prefer to avoid injections.

ARE GLP-1S FOR ME?

GLP-1 medications can be valuable tools within a comprehensive weight management approach, but they work best when integrated thoughtfully with the lifestyle changes we've discussed. Consider GLP-1s if you've been implementing calorie restriction and regular physical activity for several months but are struggling with persistent hunger, portion control, or weight loss plateaus despite consistent efforts. These medications are particularly helpful for people who find that intense appetite and cravings undermine their ability to maintain the caloric deficit needed for fat loss, or for those who have successfully lost weight in the past but struggle with long-term maintenance due to appetite regulation.

However, GLP-1s are not a substitute for developing sustainable eating habits and should be viewed as facilitators rather than replacements for lifestyle change. The most successful approach involves using the appetite-suppressing effects of these medications as an opportunity to practice and establish healthier portion sizes, meal timing, and food choices—essentially learning what appropriate hunger and satiety feel like while applying the Cholesterol Down Plan, building the habits that will support long-term success. If you're considering GLP-1 therapy, discuss with your healthcare provider whether you're a suitable candidate based on your BMI, health conditions, previous weight loss attempts, and commitment to making concurrent lifestyle modifications. Remember that these medications work best as part of a comprehensive plan that includes the calorie management and physical activity strategies outlined in these pages, not as stand-alone solutions.

GLP-1 CAUTION

Like all drugs, there are side effects. Many people initially experience GI side effects, particularly nausea, diarrhea, constipation, and vomiting. A recent study[9] found that 6 in 10 people who started the drugs quit before they saw any benefits because of these side effects. While the GI side effects tend to dissipate after a few weeks, they can substantially impact the quality of life until then.

The drugs are also ridiculously expensive—about $1,000 per month without insurance at the time of writing. If you are interested in taking these drugs but can't afford them, there are several strategies to explore: work with your healthcare provider to document medical necessity for insurance coverage (particularly if you have diabetes, prediabetes, or obesity-related health conditions), check manufacturer websites for patient assistance programs and discount coupons that can significantly reduce costs, consider starting with older GLP-1 medications like liraglutide that may have better insurance coverage. Some employers are also beginning to cover these medications as part of comprehensive wellness programs. While the price should decrease dramatically once patents expire and generic versions come to market, these immediate options may provide more accessible pathways to treatment.

Regarding safety, these new drugs have a strong safety profile based on available data, but human studies are only about five years old. This means the long-term effects are not yet fully understood.

CHOOSE YOUR DIET WISELY FOR MAXIMUM CHOLESTEROL REDUCTION

Make no mistake, if heart health is your goal, the amount of calories that you consume is important. You could still reduce daily calorie intake by eating an artery-clogging diet of French fries, burgers, and soda, or you can restrict calories by eating a heart-healthy plant-based diet. The point being that *if you are after cholesterol reduction,* the foods you eat that make up the diet will make a difference *even if you are losing weight.* Eating the recommended foods in the Cholesterol Down Plan already puts you on the road to sourcing calories from cholesterol-fighting foods. Just top them off with other nutritious foods to round out your daily calorie intake. Eating less, losing weight, and keeping it off: all of it requires you to make changes. As tough as calorie restriction can be, one small step at a time makes the impossible possible.

Ten Tips to Help You Eat Fewer Calories

1. If you are counting calories, consider using a calorie counting app on your phone to streamline the process. Apps such as SnapCalorie, MyFitnessPal, and Cronometer offer features such as AI-powered photo recognition to estimate caloric content from pictures, extensive food databases, barcode scanning, and meal-planning tools that can make tracking significantly easier than manual calculation.
2. Consider using a scale. Monitoring your body weight—once a week, at the same time of day, using the same scale, wearing the same clothes (or no clothes at all)—is a great way to maintain focus on your goals and keep yourself accountable.
3. Consider keeping a food journal. The simple task of keeping track of the calories and portion sizes of what you eat as well as the situations surrounding your food consumption is a helpful tool for staying on track and self-analyzing your personal eating habits.
4. Remove all high-calorie foods from your home environment. If you just know you will consume that entire quart of super yummy chocolate chip cookie dough ice cream, then don't have it in your freezer.
5. Substitute. Substituting healthy low-calorie foods for the high-calorie or high-fat foods that you typically eat is the most painless way to eat fewer calories. For example, try air-popped popcorn with butter spray and a dash of salt instead of the usual butter-soaked, salty popcorn; try fat-free whipped topping instead of whipped cream; enjoy thin-sliced whole grain bread instead of giant-sized hunks of white bread; eat reduced-fat peanut butter in lieu of regular.
6. Don't drink your calories! Did you know that soda and other sugar-sweetened beverages such as fruit drinks are the most consumed beverages in the U.S.—and the leading source of added sugars in our diets? Nix the soda and sugar-sweetened drinks in favor of calorie-free liquids.
7. Eat more natural foods that are filling. Foods high in volume, like fruits, vegetables, and soups, are low in calories and can

help you feel full. Vegetables like leafy greens, cucumbers, broccoli, and bell peppers are excellent low-calorie filler foods due to their high fiber and water content, along with fruits such as berries, apples, and watermelon that provide natural sweetness and satiety. Protein-rich options like egg whites, Greek yogurt, lean fish, and chicken breast offer high satiety per calorie, while foods like clear broths, air-popped popcorn, and large salads can help you feel full on fewer total calories.

8. Focus on mindful eating. Mindful eating means taking time to savor every bite and truly enjoy the eating experience. Sit at the table with no television or screens and concentrate on the aroma, texture, and flavor of food. Becoming more mindful when eating also helps you become more in touch with your body's signals of hunger and fullness.
9. Beware of restaurants! We love restaurants, with research indicating that most Americans, approximately 75 percent, dine out, order takeout, or get delivery from restaurants at least once a week.[10] The problem is the massive portion sizes served up: the average entrée clocks in at 674 calories; side dish, 260; salad almost 500 calories; specialty beverage, 418; and dessert, 429.[11] Controlling portions is essential to weight loss success. Consider sharing meals or taking half your meal home in a doggy bag.
10. Many people struggle to lose even a few pounds despite their best efforts, resulting in feelings of shame and low self-esteem. If you've tried sustainable lifestyle changes but find yourself constantly battling hunger, cravings, or persistent "food noise"—those intrusive thoughts about food that dominate your day—GLP-1 medications may be worth discussing with your healthcare provider. People who have succeeded with these medications report that the feelings of fullness and reduced hunger finally allowed them to implement the healthy habits they'd been trying to maintain. Remember that overweight and obesity can be medically treated when lifestyle changes alone prove insufficient, and there's no shame in seeking medical support for a complex health condition.

The proof that a reduced calorie plan incorporating the recommended Cholesterol Down foods is the most effective diet to promote healthy weight loss and dramatically lower LDL cholesterol has been demonstrated in a recent meta-analysis.[12] Statisticians analyzed the results from 121 randomized, controlled clinical trials with almost 22,000 overweight or obese participants, comparing the effects of 14 popular diets on markers of cardiovascular disease risk. After six months on the diets, all participants lost weight. However, the reduction in LDL cholesterol varied dramatically. This meta-analysis demonstrates a crucial point about calorie restriction: the quality of your calories determines whether weight loss improves or harms your cardiovascular health. The striking contrast between diet outcomes reveals why popular weight-loss diets often fail to deliver lasting health benefits. While the South Beach Diet's dramatic 20-pound weight loss might seem appealing, the accompanying LDL *increase* demonstrates how the wrong food choices during calorie restriction can actually worsen cardiovascular risk. In contrast, while all participants lost weight regardless of diet type, only those following heart-healthy eating patterns like the Portfolio diet achieved the dual benefit of weight loss plus dramatic LDL reduction. This reinforces why the Cholesterol Down approach emphasizes specific cholesterol-lowering foods during calorie restriction—ensuring that every pound lost also moves you closer to optimal heart health rather than compromising it.

The basis of the Cholesterol Down Plan is the concept of natural combination therapy—the safe, nonpharmacological approach for slashing cholesterol. Add in daily calorie restriction to your arsenal of LDL-lowering steps outlined in this book and watch your cholesterol plummet.

CALORIE RESTRICTION TOOLS ON THE INTERNET

For more information on how to reduce your caloric intake healthfully, I refer you to the following resources.

National Heart Lung and Blood Institute Body Mass Index Calculator (www.nhlbi.nih.gov/health/educational/lose_wt/BMI/bmicalc.htm)

WEBFCE Body Roundness Index (BRI) Calculator (https://webfce.com/bri-calculator)

American Cancer Society Calorie Counter (www.cancer.org/cancer/risk-prevention/diet-physical-activity/eat-healthy/calorie-counter-calculator.html)

National Heart Lung and Blood Institute Waist Measurement Instructions (www.nhlbi.nih.gov/health/educational/lose_wt/risk.htm)

SnapCalorie Calorie Counting App (www.snapcalorie.com)

MyFitnessPal Calorie tracking app (www.myfitnesspal.com)

Cronometer Nutrition Tracking App (www.cronometer.com)

VeryWellFit Walking Calorie Calculator (www.verywellfit.com/walking-calories-burned-per-minute-3887138) (www.verywellfit.com/measure-walking-speed-3435745)

CHAPTER 13

Step 10: Walk

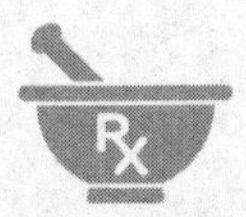

Walk for 30 minutes every day.

Dare I mention the e-word? Am I just another health professional going on and on with the mantra that exercise is good for you? The answer is a resounding yes! The tenth and final Cholesterol Down step is not a food or a supplement but a daily exercise prescription. Walking is one of the safest, simplest, most inexpensive, and most significant cholesterol-improving strategies you can adopt to complete your daily attack on LDL cholesterol. Walking offers myriad physical and mental health benefits and can be done by people of all ages and fitness levels.[1] So get your sneakers on, get ready, get set, and start to walk your cholesterol down!

Debi's Story

Debi W., age forty-three
Pre: Total cholesterol: 274 mg/dL; LDL cholesterol: 179 mg/dL
Post: Total cholesterol: 230 mg/dL; LDL cholesterol: 145 mg/dL

19 percent reduction in LDL cholesterol

Debi is a speech pathologist as well as an active, healthy wife and mother of three. She has had a longtime history of

abnormally high cholesterol as well as a close relative that had a heart attack at a very early age. Her cholesterol levels were so high that her concerned cardiologist prescribed one statin drug after another in an effort to bring her cholesterol down to normal. By the time she came to see me, she had tried five different cholesterol-lowering medications (four statins and one cholesterol absorption blocker) but unfortunately had intolerable side effects from all of them. Thus, Debi came to me seeking a nonpharmaceutical approach to lowering her cholesterol. Debi tells her experience with the Cholesterol Down Plan here.

I am a busy mother of three, in my early forties, and I try to live a healthy lifestyle of diet and exercise. My family has a history of heart disease on both sides, including an uncle who had a severe heart attack at age thirty-two, with three young children, that put him on disability since that time. I have always been concerned about my health and have known about my high levels of cholesterol, which were always in the abnormal ranges (especially my LDLs) for many years. Various doctors have made numerous suggestions, and I finally relented and started on a statin drug. I immediately had severe muscle pain and was ordered off the drug. Another doctor suggested I take a lower dose and on alternate days. This did not alter the side effects. I have taken four different statin drugs with the same results, and Zetia as well, with the same side effects. I tried to persevere, because my levels definitely dropped, but the side effects were unbearable.

I heard about Dr. Janet Brill's plan, and after speaking with her, I decided it was definitely worth a shot. At first it felt like a lot of food (which was good, because you are never hungry!), but by week two it became second nature. The daily walking was easy and a wonderful addition to my lifestyle. I felt great and was excited to see what would happen with my labs. Well, after just four weeks, my LDL dropped significantly (almost 20 percent), as well as my triglycerides and total cholesterol. Even my cardiologist was impressed. I am going to continue with this program, and hopefully my numbers will continue to drop to normal levels. This is definitely going to be a lifestyle change, but if I feel good and have no side effects, the results speak for themselves.

Most important, this is something I will teach my children so they can understand the importance of good nutrition and the various foods that can have a positive impact on your health throughout your life. Thank you, Dr. Brill!

COUCH POTATO NATION

If you're not an exercise enthusiast, you are not alone—in fact, you are in the majority. According to the Centers for Disease Control and Prevention (CDC), we are a nation of inactive people. This is not surprising considering that 74 percent of us are classified as overweight and that lack of exercise goes hand in hand with excess poundage. How popular is it to do no exercise whatsoever? The CDC reports that 25 percent of us are "sedentary," meaning we move very little—we perform no leisure-time activities that expend calories such as walking, gardening, or golf. Some of us report getting some exercise—but apparently not enough. In fact, according to the CDC, only 24.2 percent of U.S. adults meet the guidelines for both aerobic and muscle-strengthening activities, meaning more than three-quarters of Americans do not get enough physical activity to promote better health.[2] Let's face it: we are truly a nation of couch potatoes.

"So what?" you may be thinking. Well, think again. The message from the nation's heart health experts is clear: physical inactivity is a *major* risk factor for heart disease.

Statistics of a Sedentary Society

- Physical inactivity ranks up there with smoking, high blood pressure, and high cholesterol as a major risk factor for heart disease.

- People who are insufficiently active have a 20–30 percent increased risk of death compared to people who are sufficiently active.
- About 35 percent of deaths from heart disease are due to physical inactivity.
- Twice as many Americans are as inactive as those who smoke cigarettes.
- The combination of physical inactivity, overweight, and obesity is considered a major contributor to overall healthcare costs in the United States, with estimates suggesting it accounts for approximately 27 percent of total healthcare expenditures nationwide.

Sources: Marjolein Duijvestijn et al., "Impact of Physical Activity on Healthcare Costs: A Systematic Review," BMC Health Services Research 23, no. 1 (2023), https://doi.org/10.1186/s12913-023-09556-8; "Physical Activity Fact Sheet," World Health Organization, www.who.int/news-room/fact-sheets/detail/physical-activity.

CHOOSING AN EXERCISE ROUTINE THAT'S RIGHT FOR YOU

You have decided to start an exercise program, so you turn to the experts for guidance. Exercise for twenty minutes, three times a week. No, make that thirty minutes on most days of the week. Better yet, make that a full hour every day. No, ten minutes here and ten minutes there will do. No wonder people are confused! Although the seemingly contradictory exercise recommendation messages can be frustrating, the straight answer about how much is enough is that it depends on your goals. If weight loss is your primary goal, then you may need to exercise more than someone exercising to obtain other health benefits. That's because to lose weight, you need to burn more calories than you consume. In a society where it is all too easy to eat an excessive amount of calories, performing a large amount of calorie-burning exercise daily will offset the excess calorie intake and either promote weight loss or prevent further weight gain.

For cholesterol management and disease prevention, the Cholesterol Down Plan includes a goal of thirty minutes of continuous walking every day. If you haven't been exercising regularly, then start out slowly with modest increments and build up from there. A starting schedule would include twenty minutes of walking two to three days a week, progressing to five days, then seven days, then increasing walking time to thirty minutes. Do not worry about the pace until you can complete the full exercise prescription: seven days, thirty minutes. After you achieve that goal, focus on speeding up your pace, because faster is healthier. If this exercise prescription is simply not doable in your mind, you can adjust the walking time to fewer days per week. A study, conducted over ten years and published in *JAMA*, has found that people who took 8,000 or more steps on just one or two days of the week had a 14.9 percent lower risk of death compared to people who were sedentary.[3]

GETTING MOTIVATED

Do most of us not exercise because the recommendations are too conflicting? Or because we are much more inclined to spend our time working, reading, watching TV, scrolling social media, and, all too often, eating at the same time? The most frequent reasons my patients share with me for why they don't exercise are "I don't have the time" followed by "I don't enjoy it," "I was never athletic," "It's a waste of time," and "It's too expensive to join a club." The underlying problem is that people perceive the costs of exercise as too great relative to the rewards. The truth is, we like instant gratification more than long-term benefits, such as preventing chronic disease. This is why it is important to give yourself tangible rewards, such as walking with a good friend or listening to your favorite music during your walk, to help you adopt exercise as a daily habit.

EIGHT IMPORTANT REASONS TO EXERCISE

1. Walking lowers LDL cholesterol. You are reading this book and trying this plan with the goal of lowering your "bad" LDL cholesterol. Walking just thirty minutes a day is a simple and highly effective strategy for cholesterol reduction and has been proven to effectively cut LDL cholesterol levels in both men and women.[4]

2. Not exercising is as unhealthy as smoking cigarettes. You may vehemently oppose the idea of smoking cigarettes for fear of cancer but not think twice about being totally sedentary. Consider that the American Heart Association lists lack of physical activity as a major risk factor for heart disease, *equal in risk* to cigarette smoking, high blood pressure, or high cholesterol.[5]

3. Exercise prevents diabetes. We have an epidemic of type 2 diabetes (the kind associated with overweight and obesity) in this country. A review of numerous clinical trials investigating the role of physical activity in preventing diabetes has unequivocally demonstrated that a moderate aerobic exercise program can cut your risk of developing this dreadful disease. Walking briskly for more than 150 minutes per week was sufficient to protect study participants.[6]

4. Exercise helps you live longer. People who are fitter do live longer and better. This is especially true when looking at heart disease risk. A study published in the prestigious medical journal *Archives of Internal Medicine* has shown that a workout a day can add nearly four years to your life. A sample of over 5,000 participants taken from the noted Framingham Heart Study found that people who engaged in moderate exercise (walking for thirty minutes at least five days a week) lived about 1.3 to 1.5 more years than less active individuals. More intense exercisers (running for thirty minutes at least five days a week) lived even longer (3.5 to 3.7 more years) compared to their sedentary counterparts.[7]

Ten Ways to Promote Regular Exercise

1. Consider tracking your steps on your cell phone. Record the number of daily steps you take and try to increase that amount weekly, with an eventual goal of 10,000 steps per day. (For more information on walking apps, see "Walking on the Internet" on page 206.)
2. Draw up an exercise schedule one week at a time and post the schedule on the refrigerator. Be systematic; do not let anything interfere with the time allotted for exercise. Cross off each day that you accomplish your goal. At the end of the week, give yourself a reward such as a steam or sauna bath, a massage, or a soy latte.
3. Put a treadmill in front of the TV. Only allow yourself to watch your favorite show if you walk on the treadmill.
4. Keep an extra pair of running or walking shoes in the trunk of your car and seize the moment. Do a few laps around the soccer field while waiting to pick up the kids at school or during a soccer game. Walk along the beach rather than sunbathe. Walk rather than ride the golf cart when playing golf, and carry your own clubs.
5. If you plan to exercise in the early morning and just can't seem to stop turning off the alarm and going back to sleep, prepare the night before: put the alarm clock across the room so you have to get out of bed to turn it off, set out your exercise clothes, and have an automatic coffeemaker brew your coffee so the smell of fresh-brewed coffee can entice you out of bed.
6. Hire a personal trainer. This is well worth the money, because if you make an appointment and you have to pay for the session, you are much more likely to go. Make sure you have great rapport with your trainer; if you like his or her personality, you will be much more likely to attend. (For information on finding a reliable personal trainer, see "Walking on the Internet" on page 206.)

7. Learn and practice time management. Pencil in exercise sessions on your calendar as if they were dental appointments, so you will be more likely to follow through with the exercise session and respect it as you would any other commitment.
8. Go back to an old American pastime and take an after-dinner stroll every night. Set aside thirty minutes to walk off dinner and relax. No distractions, just a thirty-minute period for reflection and winding down the day.
9. Organize a morning exercise group or join a walking club. If you are accountable only to yourself, it's easier to find excuses not to exercise. If you are accountable to another person, you have a greater responsibility to show up.
10. Buy gadgets that make exercise more fun, such as a heart monitor or a GPS watch. Or walk to your favorite thirty-minute playlist and don't stop until the last song ends. Listen to your audiobook chapter or perhaps your favorite podcast on your device.

5. **Exercise reduces risk of contracting breast and colon cancer.** Scientists at the University of Southern California Medical School found that the risk of getting breast cancer was 35 percent lower in women with a history of regular exercise. Exercise also dramatically helps survival in women diagnosed with breast cancer. According to data from the long-running Harvard Nurses' Health Study (tracking 122,000 nurses for eighteen years), walking 3–5 hours per week cut risk of death by 50 percent. And a meta-analysis of nineteen studies clearly demonstrates that physical activity lowers the risk of contracting colon and rectal cancer.[8]

6. **Exercise will enhance your golden years.** As we age, we lose muscle mass and our fitness level severely declines. Low strength and fitness levels in the elderly frequently equate to frailty and loss of independence. Exercising into our golden

years is an ideal strategy for attenuating the inevitable decline in fitness that comes with age.[9]

7. **Exercise is good for the brain and will dramatically cut your risk of dementia.** For more than thirty-five years, Swedish researchers monitored the exercise habits of nearly 1,500 elderly patients. Those patients who had engaged in physical activity at least twice a week from midlife onward had a 50 percent lower risk of developing dementia and a 60 percent lower chance of developing Alzheimer's disease compared to their non-exercising counterparts.[10]

8. **Exercise saves you money.** If the myriad health benefits are not enough to get you off the couch, perhaps a strong financial incentive will motivate you to tie up those laces. A study of nearly 7,000 men spanning nineteen years found that fit men reduced their medical bills by 46 percent compared to their sedentary counterparts. What's more, those men who started an exercise program and shaped up lowered their chances of being hospitalized by 42 percent.[11]

EXERCISE AS MEDICINE

Why make the effort to get up earlier (ugh) and leave the comfort of your warm cozy bed for a stroll around the block in the dead of winter? Why head for the treadmill instead of the computer? First, once you finish that walk, the endorphins flowing through your brain give you a natural high. Second, getting the blood flowing through your veins truly makes us feel more alive. Third, getting more physically fit will help you to live better in all areas of your life. And fourth, taking a daily stroll has the power to help ward off cardiovascular disease (heart attacks and stroke), diabetes, breast and colon cancer, osteoporosis, depression, and Alzheimer's disease as well as reduce the risk of erectile dysfunction in older men. Miraculous or what?

Did you know that one simple lifestyle change—getting up and walking for a mere thirty minutes a day—will dramatically cut your chances of dying? There is a saying among health and fitness professionals: "Exercise is medicine." If there were a daily pill that helped you to lose weight, age more gracefully, ward off chronic disease, prevent dementia, depression, and impotence, plus lower your cholesterol (with no side effects except a sense of euphoria) and was virtually free, wouldn't you take it? Well, that miracle pill exists, and it is called exercise. So I ask you, why not make exercise a daily priority?

Physical inactivity is one of the top three adverse life habits that, according to the National Cholesterol Education Program, must be addressed in the prevention of heart disease. The other two are an artery-clogging diet and being classified as overweight. NCEP's therapeutic lifestyle changes include instituting a therapeutic diet to help lower LDL cholesterol and engaging in physical activity on a daily basis.[12] NCEP also emphasizes the importance of weight loss as a strategy for cholesterol management; it's a well-known fact that exercise is the cornerstone of all effective weight management programs.

Women and Walking: A Proven LDL Reduction Strategy

A meta-analysis of twenty-one studies investigated changes in blood cholesterol following walking interventions among women with overweight and obesity (approximately 1,100 subjects). The results showed that the walkers had a significant drop in LDL cholesterol, an average decline of 7 mg/dL compared to non-walkers. (Most study participants walked approximately 30 minutes per day at a moderate intensity.) The takeaway is that daily walking reduces LDL cholesterol levels, and it is a safe and effective cardiovascular intervention for weight management. The research confirmed that a minimum of four weeks of walking exercise helps normalize LDL cholesterol in women with overweight.

Source: A. M. Ballard et al., "The Effects of Exclusive Walking on Lipids and Lipoproteins in Women with Overweight and Obesity: A Systematic Review and Meta-Analysis," *American Journal of Health Promotion* 36, no. 2 (2022): 328–339.

WALKING, A GREAT FORM OF AEROBIC EXERCISE

Walking is the most popular form of exercise in the United States. Walking is safe and easy and requires no special equipment (other than a good pair of walking shoes), no fancy clothing, and no expensive gym membership. It can be done just about anywhere and is a healthful type of aerobic exercise. Aerobic exercise—*aerobic* literally means "using oxygen"—consists of activities such as walking, running, biking, and swimming that use the large muscle groups on a repetitive basis for a sustained period of time. Unlike aerobic exercise, anaerobic exercise can be fueled "without oxygen." Examples of anaerobic exercise include weight training, sprinting, and sports involving short bursts of high-power activity such as tennis. All exercise is good for you, but it is the aerobic types that are most beneficial for making positive changes to your cardiovascular health profile—raising HDL and lowering LDL cholesterol—and your blood vessels. Blood vessel health reflects cardiovascular health.

Walk Your Weight and Your Cholesterol Down

In my own research at the University of Miami, I put 56 women with overweight on a heart-healthy calorie-restricted weight-loss diet. I divided them into three groups: no exercise, walking thirty minutes a day, or walking sixty minutes a day. At the end of the twelve-week program, participants in all groups lost an average of eleven pounds. Interestingly, only the walkers made a significant dent in their LDL cholesterol, dropping an average of 10 percent! Plus, only the walkers showed a significant reduction in the amount of belly fat, the stubborn fat that collects around the middle and is associated with the significant risk of developing health problems such as diabetes and heart disease.

I also found that when people were responsible to another party (me) and to meeting up with their friends, they walked more frequently and for longer periods. What's more, they reported that the simple task of walking with their friends made the walking a pleasure rather than an exercise chore.

Thus, my research showed that a twelve-week walking program (either thirty or sixty minutes five times per week at a self-selected pace) not only lowered the subjects' centralized body fat stores but cut LDL cholesterol and improved fitness as well.

Source: Janet Bond Brill, "A Comparison of Different Exercise Prescriptions Combined with a Low-Fat Ad Libitum Diet: Effects on Weight Loss, Health-Related Variables and Psychological Well-Being in Premenopausal Overweight Women," PhD dissertation, University of Miami, Coral Gables, Florida, May 2001, https://scholarship.miami.edu/esploro/outputs/doctoral/A-comparison-of-different-exercise-prescriptions/991031447942402976.

EXERCISE FOR A HEALTHY HEART

Exercise Makes the Heart Stronger

Exercise provides an arsenal of artillery in the fight against cardiovascular disease. Regular aerobic exercise, such as walking, favorably modifies heart disease risk factors such as high blood pressure, diabetes, and living with overweight, in addition to having a positive effect on factors directly involved with the process of atherosclerosis (LDL and HDL cholesterol and blood vessel dynamics). What's more, exercise training makes the heart stronger by improving the ability of the heart muscle to contract, improving the heart's electrical stability, and increasing the supply of oxygen and nutrients to the heart muscle.

UP WITH THE "GOOD" HDL, DOWN WITH THE "BAD" LDL

When it comes to exercise and cholesterol, the general scientific consensus has been that a regular program of aerobic exercise raises the level of "good" HDL cholesterol. Most studies have shown that the greater the volume of aerobic exercise performed, the greater the rise in your level of HDL. An emerging body of evidence shows that LDL cholesterol is also positively affected by a program of regular aerobic exercise: it is significantly decreased. But just how much can exercise cut LDL cholesterol? A meta-analysis of ninety-five studies performed decades ago concluded that exercise training leads to a 10.1 percent reduction in LDL cholesterol.[13]

A meta-analysis of twenty-five studies found that walking exercise specifically decreases LDL cholesterol by approximately 5–6 percent, regardless of whether participants lost weight.[14] Perhaps the strong LDL-lowering effect of walking is why walking is associated with a longer life. The Honolulu Heart Program, which followed 707 retired men for a period of twelve years, revealed that the risk of death among the men who walked the least (less than one mile a day) was double that of those men who walked one to two miles per day.[15]

WALKING ALSO CUTS RISK OF STROKE

Stroke is another common form of cardiovascular disease and is a major killer—the third leading cause of death in the United States. (Heart disease and cancer are number one and number two.) Merely walking or biking to or from work for up to twenty-nine minutes per day was enough to cut risk of stroke by 8 percent compared to non-exercisers and by 11 percent for those logging in thirty minutes or more on their way to work, according to a Finnish study of more than 47,000 subjects who were followed for nineteen years.[16] High levels of exercise such as running, swimming, or heavy gardening can reduce your risk even further. This is the first study to clearly prove a distinct inverse relationship between physical activity and risk of any type of stroke—meaning the more exercise you do, the lower your chances of having a stroke.

EXERCISE PLUS DIET PRODUCES MAXIMUM LDL REDUCTION

Exercise is a helpful and necessary addition to a lifestyle designed to cut cholesterol. That's the message from a classic study out of the Stanford Center for Research in Disease Prevention.[17] Scientists investigated the effects of aerobic exercise plus an NCEP Step 2 diet on LDL cholesterol in men and women with high initial levels (over 125 mg/dL). After one year, the greatest decline in LDL cholesterol (14.5 mg/dL for women and 20 mg/dL for men) was observed in the combination diet-plus-exercise group, compared to negligible reductions in both the exercise-only and diet-only groups.

EXERCISE PLUS DIET MAKES YOUR STATIN DRUG WORK BETTER

Don't fool yourself into believing that popping your statin pill will allow you to shelve your athletic shoes, sit back on the couch, and continue to eat the same artery-clogging foods without paying the price down the road. Combining diet and exercise with a statin drug prevents heart attacks more effectively than medication alone. That was the finding in a University of Texas Medical School study of 409 people already diagnosed with heart disease.[18] Subjects were divided into three groups: the poor-treatment group (no special diet, exercise, or drugs), the moderate-treatment group (either an American Heart Association diet with a statin drug or a strict low-fat diet alone), and the maximal-treatment group (a statin drug, a strict low-fat diet, and aerobic exercise thirty minutes or more four to five days a week). After five years, the maximal-treatment group came out way ahead, with only 7 percent having suffered an "event," meaning a heart attack, stroke, or other cardiac-related incident. Compare this to subjects in the moderate-treatment group, who were three times as likely to suffer an event, or in the poor-treatment group, who fared the worst—31 percent experienced an event.

AEROBIC EXERCISE AND YOUR HEALTH

How Does Aerobic Exercise Prevent Heart Disease?

Decades of research demonstrate that regular aerobic exercise, whether through walking, swimming, cycling, or running, provides remarkable protection against heart disease by improving multiple aspects of cardiovascular function. Regular aerobic exercise fights LDL and heart disease on the following fronts:

Method of Attack #1. Walking boosts LDL resistance to oxidation. Spanish researchers compared the LDL of aerobically trained subjects with sedentary subjects and found that regular aerobic exercise significantly strengthened the ability of LDL to resist oxidation, thus protecting against atherosclerosis in the arteries.[19] Another study out of Finland had similar findings. Finnish researchers had 104 men and women follow an exercise program (mostly walking) for ten months. Not only did the subjects' LDL cholesterol drop by an average of about 11 percent, but HDL increased and the antioxidant potential of LDL was strengthened by a huge 23 percent. Another bonus: the participants lost an average of five pounds, and their body fat declined an average of 3 percent.[20]

Why does walking prevent oxidation? Oxidation is a process that involves three factors: the enemy—free radicals (highly unstable molecules that attack your cells); the victim—LDL particles that are highly vulnerable to attack (the small, dense type is most susceptible to oxidation); and the defenders—the body's antioxidant defense team that protects against the destructive free radicals. The antioxidant defenders come from foods you eat and the antioxidant chemicals that your cells manufacture. Here's where exercise comes in. Research indicates that aerobic exercise increases the heart's production of an antioxidant enzyme called superoxide dismutase, a key defender against free radical damage.[21]

Method of Attack #2. Walking changes the size and shape of LDL particles in your bloodstream, beneficially altering them so that they are less dangerous. A study out of Duke University provided data to support this claim.[22] The eight-month trial involving men and women experiencing overweight showed that walking twelve miles per week was enough to promote the healthful changes. A more recent series of meta-analyses from exercise training studies[23] supports the conclusion that regular exercise changes the size and shape of LDL cholesterol particles to a less dangerous type.

How does walking have such a pronounced effect on LDL? Regular aerobic exercise trains the muscle and fat cells to produce more of an enzyme called lipoprotein lipase (LPL). You may already know this all-important enzyme as the body's key fat-burning chemical. Enhanced levels of LPL have two important actions related to cholesterol metabolism: a higher level of LPL activity lowers the amount of circulating VLDL (the parent of LDL) and chylomicrons (cholesterol-containing balls of fat derived from intestinal cells that head toward the liver), and the makeup of the VLDL particles is altered (they contain less triglyceride), resulting in VLDL particles that eventually are transformed into enlarged LDL particles, which, as we've already seen, are less likely to enter the inner layer of artery walls and contribute to plaque buildup and atherosclerosis.[24] (The dangerous, small, dense LDL particles arise from larger, fluffier, and more triglyceride-filled VLDL precursors.)

Method of Attack #3. If you are someone with overweight and your cholesterol level is worrisome, you need to lose weight and exercise thirty minutes or more most days of the week to manage your cholesterol problem and lower your risk of heart disease. Maintaining a healthy body weight is crucial because there is a strong connection between excess weight and high LDL cholesterol. As your body fat goes up, your liver naturally produces more LDL cholesterol. Lose weight, and your LDL goes down.

Where you store your fat affects your likelihood of developing not only heart disease but also diabetes and high blood pressure. People who tend to gather fat around the middle (potbellies) are at far greater risk for metabolic problems than those who accumulate fat in other areas such as the hips or thighs. Even a small amount of fat in the abdominal area is worse for you than a large amount in the lower body. Not exercising increases your chances of accumulating belly fat, but incorporating a walking program will help alleviate this problem while lowering your LDL cholesterol. As noted previously, my own research showed that walking trims dangerous deep abdominal fat and targets LDL cholesterol. Some researchers think that exercise improves the body's ability to utilize insulin. This in turn increases the activity of LDL receptors on the liver, which enhances clearance of LDL from the bloodstream, subsequently lowering LDL levels.[25]

Method of Attack #4. The pace of exercise is another factor that affects heart health. Imagine the flow of blood through the arteries as water flowing down a river. The branch points in the arterial river where the flow of blood is disturbed are the areas most prone to clogging up with plaque. The disturbed blood flow—such as where the carotid arteries leading up to the brain branch off—irritates the delicate cells lining the arterial wall, causing inflammation. However, brisk walks speed up the flow of blood through the arteries, which reduces clogging and inflammation and therefore helps prevent the atherosclerotic process.

SHEAR STRESS IS GOOD STRESS

Bumping up the intensity of your workouts is beneficial for the blood vessels because it increases what is termed "shear stress," or a substantial increase in the speed of blood flowing through the blood vessels. Increasing shear stress for an extended period, such as when you take a brisk walk, prompts the cells lining arteries to increase production of their own anti-inflammatory chemicals, particularly nitric oxide.[26] Nitric oxide promotes dilation of the vessels' interior diameters, which helps prevent clogging and lessens the chance of a heart attack. Nitric oxide also inhibits sprouting of the adhesion molecules that attract immune system cells to perpetuate atherosclerosis. What's more, nitric oxide suppresses a host of inflammatory chemicals, increases the activity of antioxidant enzymes, and lessens the ability of platelets to congregate and stick together—effects that hinder the formation of deadly blood clots and potentially protect you against having a heart attack.[27]

Pick Up the Pace for Maximum Heart Protection

Is faster better, or is a leisurely stroll just as cardioprotective? In the famous Harvard School of Public Health Study that began in 1986, researchers followed 44,452 male health professionals over a twelve-year period and found that those who exercised at high intensity experienced significantly reduced cardiovascular risk. Men who ran for at least an hour a week (at 6 mph or faster) were 42 percent less likely to succumb to heart disease than non-runners. Brisk walkers (at least 3 mph for at least thirty minutes per day) were 18 percent less likely to develop heart disease than non-walkers. Low-intensity walkers did not gain any heart benefits. A study conducted out of the United Kingdom thirty-six years later followed 78,500 people over seven years and found that individuals who took up to 10,000 steps per day had a significantly lower risk of death and cardiovascular disease compared to non-walkers. Those who walked at a faster pace had additional health benefits.

Sources: Mihaela Tanasescu et al., "Exercise Type and Intensity in Relation to Coronary Heart Disease in Men," *JAMA* 288, no. 16 (2002): 1994–2000; Borja del Pozo Cruz et al., "Prospective Associations of Daily Step Counts and Intensity With Cancer and Cardiovascular Disease Incidence and Mortality and All-Cause Mortality," *JAMA Internal Medicine* 182, no. 11 (2022): 1139–1148, doi:10.1001/jamainternmed.2022.4000.

EXERCISE REDUCES BLOOD MARKER FOR INFLAMMATION

Doctors use C-reactive protein (CRP) as a blood marker to determine if you are at risk for heart disease. High levels are indicative of an inflammatory condition; thus CRP is a powerful and accurate predictor of heart disease and stroke. CRP also contributes to the ominous buildup of plaque by shutting down the production of nitric oxide, the plaque prevention chemical discussed above. Additionally, CRP fuels the growth of adhesion molecules and increases the production and release of chemicals that attract immune system cells to the endothelial cell, thus contributing to inflammation and ultimately atherosclerosis. However, when researchers put 52 volunteers with a high initial CRP level on an individualized exercise program for six months (averaging 2.5 hours of exercise per week), their CRP levels dropped 35 percent.[28]

WALK SAFELY

If you have two or more risk factors for heart disease, make sure you get the go-ahead from your physician before beginning your walking program. You can calculate the number of risk factors you have by turning to Appendix 5, "What's Your Risk of Heart Disease?" Consulting with your doctor is also advised for sedentary individuals who are just beginning a new exercise regimen.

A five-minute warm-up period consisting of a slow walk is crucial before you begin your exercise, to get the blood flowing and to help your body adjust to the stress of exercise. Cooling down and performing a basic walker's stretching routine focusing on calves, hamstrings, and quadriceps is another segment of your exercise routine that should not be omitted. Stretching exercises performed after your muscles are all warmed up will help increase your flexibility, and flexibility is one category of physical fitness that severely declines with age.

Remember to stay hydrated—drink water before, during, and after your workout—and dress for the elements. Cold weather requires breathable layers of clothing and a hat (approximately 30 percent of body heat is lost from the head). Warm and humid weather requires light, breathable clothing as well as a hat to protect skin against damage from the sun. If the outdoor weather is severe—either extremely cold or hot and humid or with lightning present—walk indoors. If you have chest pains, feel light-headed or dizzy, or experience severe shortness of breath or pain, stop walking and immediately call your physician.

Two-Minute Post-Walking Stretching Routine

Follow your walking cool-down with some relaxed stretches. Tight, stiff muscles will benefit from controlled, comfortable stretching. These simple exercises will help increase your flexibility and possibly prevent future injuries. Remember, the stretching position should give you a feeling of tightness, never pain. Do not bounce. Gently guide your body to the point of tightness, breathe normally, and try to relax.

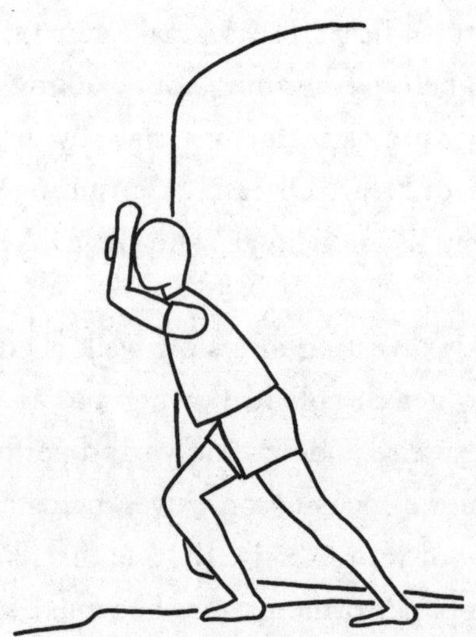

1. **Calf stretch.** Lean against a wall or tree, right leg extended backward, left leg bent. Hold for twenty seconds. Repeat stretch with opposite leg.

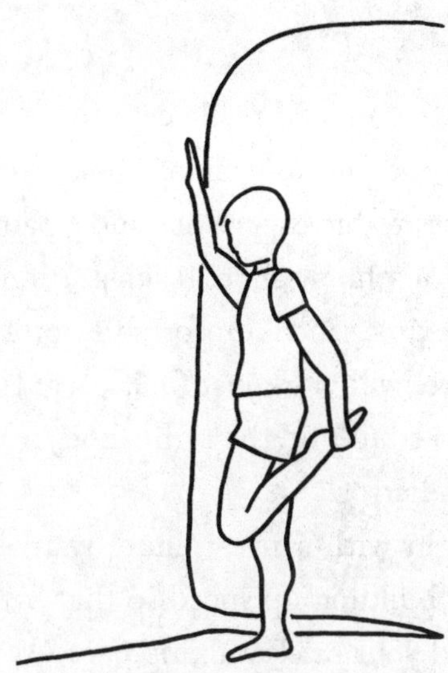

2. **Quadriceps stretch.** Place left hand against a wall. Bend right leg, grasp ankle with right hand, and gently pull. Hold for twenty seconds. Repeat stretch with opposite leg. *Note:* You can also use the opposite hand to grab the ankle. This will help keep your knees together and put less stress on the knee joint.

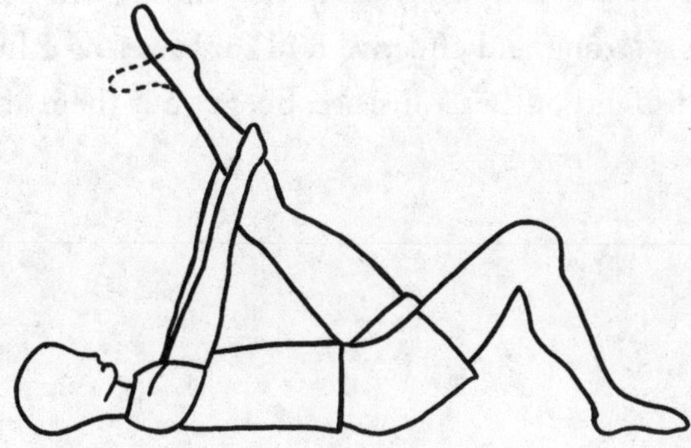

3. **Hamstring stretch.** Lie down on your back. Bend right knee, extend left leg upward, and gently pull left leg toward your chest, keeping head and neck on the floor. Hold for twenty seconds. Repeat stretch with opposite leg.

Illustrations by Eileen Eskin Brill

FILLING THE PRESCRIPTION

Walking is virtually free of charge, safe, fun, and really easy to do. The only special equipment required is a good pair of walking shoes, which can make the difference between an enjoyable experience and a painful one. Keep in mind that any good pair of athletic shoes (such as running shoes) that provide support, are flexible and comfortable, provide proper cushioning, and have a low heel will work just fine. There is no best walking shoe for everyone. You need to find the right shoe *for you,* and that often comes through trial and error.

Every walking session should begin with a five-minute warm-up, walking at a slow pace and gradually building up speed so that by the end of the warm-up you have reached your brisk walking pace. At the end of your walking session, take five more minutes to cool down, gradually returning to your initial slow pace. Cool-downs prevent bouts of dizziness that can come from abruptly stopping exercise. Be sure to finish every walking workout with a quick two-minute stretching routine.

I invite you to join those of us who have made exercise a priority in life. Regular aerobic exercise will improve your quality of life, will help you to live longer, and is a strong and effective tool for lowering LDL cholesterol and helping to fend off heart disease. So, get out there and take your daily walk!

 Cholesterol Down Walking Exercise Prescriptions

Level	Beginner*	Intermediate**	Advanced***
Walks per Week	Begin with 3, progress to 5, then to 7	7	7
Warm-Up Time	5 minutes	5 minutes	5 minutes
Minutes Walking	Begin with 20, gradually progress to 30 (only after you have reached 7 days)	30	30
Intensity	Moderate pace (as fast as possible while still able to keep a conversation going)	Brisk pace (3 mph or more)	Gradual uphill incline on treadmill (maximum 10% incline at a fast 3.5 mph or greater pace)
Cool-down Time	5 minutes	5 minutes	5 minutes
Post-exercise Stretching	2 minutes	2 minutes	2 minutes

* Beginner: For those of you who have been inactive or are recovering from an illness, your doctor may recommend that you start slowly with this exercise prescription.

** Intermediate: If you are accustomed to regular exercise and your doctor deems that you are physically fit, then your doctor may agree that this exercise prescription is for you.

*** Advanced: If you are in good shape, are accustomed to regular exercise, and are looking for a higher-intensity walking exercise prescription, this advanced uphill treadmill walking workout may be for you. On the treadmill, look for a preset gradual incline custom program workout. After your warm-up, enter a maximum of a 10 percent grade (sometimes equates with a level 10) and a fast walking pace you are comfortable with (3.5 mph or higher). Most "easy incline" workouts start at a 0 percent grade and progress up to and peak at the maximum incline (10 percent in this case) at about 75 percent through your workout (22 minutes). At this point you should be huffing and puffing and have reached the top, then it's all downhill from there!

Walking on the Internet

There is an abundance of information on the internet pertaining to health, fitness, and walking in particular. Here are some reliable sources on exercise, walking, and walking programs that I hope can help answer any additional questions you may have.

The American Heart Association's Six-Week Beginner Walking Plan (www.bu.edu/fitrec/files/2020/03/AHA-walking-plan.pdf)

American College of Sports Medicine (www.acsm.org)

The Walking Site (www.thewalkingsite.com)

Best Treadmills of 2024 Reviews (www.consumerreports.org/health/treadmills/best-treadmills-of-the-year-a6151534118)

The Best Walking Apps

StepsApp

Pacer

MapMyWalk

Argus

Fitbit

Peloton

Reliable Personal Trainer Directories

American College of Sports Medicine (www.acsm.org)

American Council on Exercise (www.acefitness.org)

National Academy of Sports Medicine (www.nasm.org)

National Strength and Conditioning Association (www.nsca-lift.org)

A Few Closing Words from Dr. Janet

Cardiovascular disease remains the leading cause of death and disability among adults in the United States and the rest of the Western world, with heart attacks as the most prevalent form. I hope you have learned from this book that death from heart disease is largely preventable, with therapeutic lifestyle changes—namely, a combination of healthy diet and exercise—as the foremost strategy for prevention. At the time of writing this revision, the scientific evidence[1] continues to be indisputable: lowering your LDL cholesterol level will help prevent cardiovascular disease, and sustaining a lower LDL level for longer is better. Will lowering your LDL cholesterol, even if just by a few points, really make a difference in your risk of heart disease? Absolutely! Reducing LDL cholesterol by as little as 15 percent and maintaining that over the long term can dramatically lessen your risk of having a heart attack.[2] That's why lowering LDL cholesterol is the thrust of the government's National Cholesterol Education Program for the prevention of heart disease.

Many patients have come to me needing to lower LDL cholesterol, yet are uncomfortable with the notion of taking statin drugs. These people are looking for a natural and healthful alternative method for lowering their "bad" cholesterol. Furthermore, they are often unaware of the new and powerful combination lifestyle therapy currently available. I have helped these people to lower their LDL cholesterol through the natural lifestyle approach that I formulated, the Cholesterol Down Plan. This simple, safe, and effective ten-step plan was designed to make it easier for individuals wishing to significantly lower their "bad" cholesterol using a drug-free lifestyle approach.

Many different foods, supplements, and exercise routines are individually effective in lowering LDL cholesterol, but I have found that my Cholesterol Down combination creates the most potent health-promoting and non-pharmaceutical strategy for lowering your "bad" cholesterol. Many of the steps in the plan are basically plain old healthy eating, with no harmful side effects or expensive prescription medications. Most of the foods on the plan can be purchased at your local supermarket. Add in a couple supplements and some walking, and you have a safe and effective natural alternative to prescription medication for lowering cholesterol.

Ideally, it is best to get in all ten steps each day. However, nobody is perfect. Checking off as many as possible, as often as possible, will surely help you in your goal of getting your LDL number where you want it to be. Good luck in following this plan—and sticking to it for life. I sincerely hope that you are successful in getting, and keeping, your cholesterol down!

To your health,

Dr. Janet Brill

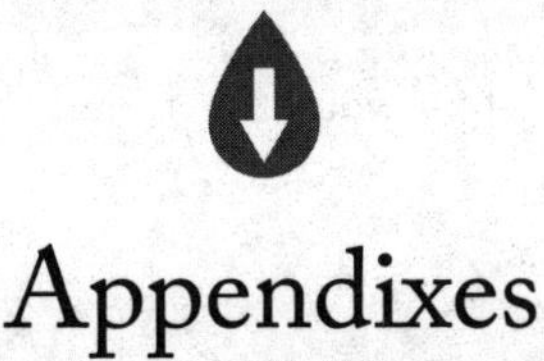

Appendixes

Appendix 1

Cholesterol Down Ten-Step Daily Checklist

Day of the week: ____________

Remember . . . the more steps you take today, the more potent the LDL cholesterol-lowering effect!

Twice a Day	Once a Day
☐ ☐ Plant sterols/stanols (CholestOff) Take 3 capsules at two separate meals ☐ ☐ Soy protein (10 grams twice a day) ☐ ☐ Psyllium Husk (Metamucil) (work up to ~3 grams a.m. and 3 grams p.m.)	☐ Oatmeal (1 bowl with added oat bran) ☐ Flaxseeds (2 tablespoons ground) ☐ Apple (one) ☐ Beans, peas, lentils (½ cup serving) ☐ Almonds (handful) ☐ Restrict daily calorie intake ☐ Walking (30 minutes, fast)

Plant sterols/stanols: Take 3 capsules of CholestOff twice a day with meals.

Soy protein: Eat 20–25 grams per day; aim for at least two servings of soy products per day.

Metamucil: Eat 3–10 grams psyllium (either 6–18 capsules or 1–2 tablespoons powder) per day, divided between 2 meals.

Oatmeal: Eat 1 cup of oatmeal or barley per day (3 grams of beta-glucan).

Flaxseeds: Eat 1–2 tablespoons of ground flaxseeds every day.

Apple: Eat one apple every day.

Beans: Eat a half cup of some type of beans, peas, or lentils every day.

Almonds: Eat 1–1½ ounces of almonds or walnuts every day or 2–3 tablespoons of almond butter.

Calorie restriction: Eat approximately 10 percent fewer calories than you typically do using whatever technique works for you (e.g., intermittent fasting, calorie counting, etc.).

Walking: Walk 30 minutes every day (preferably at a fast pace).

Appendix 2

LDL Cholesterol Progress Chart

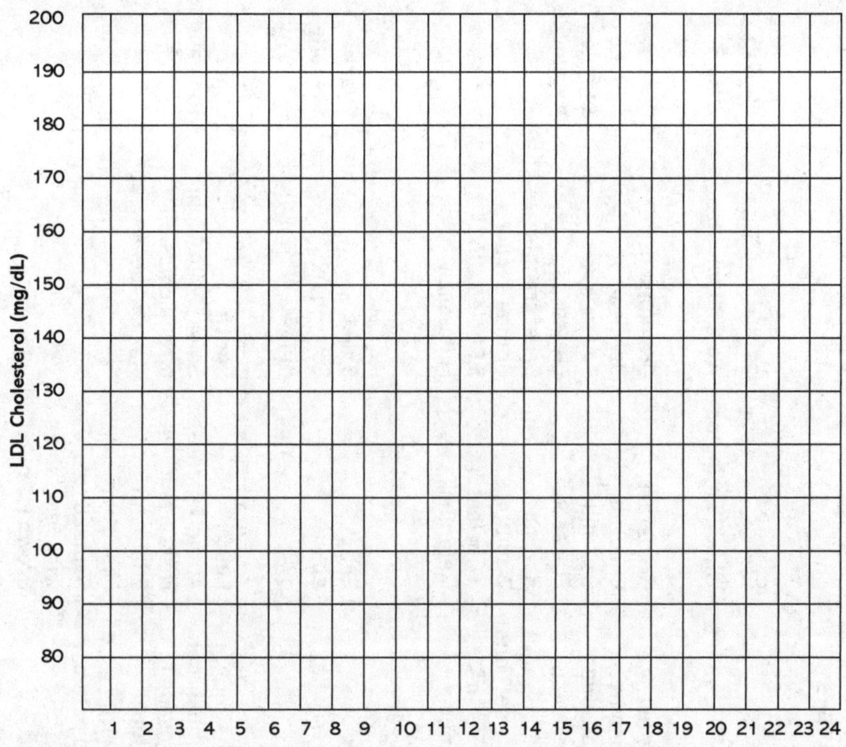

Starting LDL cholesterol (mg/dL): __________

Starting date: __________

Note: Retest at four-week intervals; use the same testing situation (i.e., fasting, same time of day, and the same laboratory).

Appendix 3

Sample Cholesterol Down Meal* and Exercise Plans

Monday	Tuesday	Wednesday	Thursday	Friday	Saturday	Sunday
Walk 30 minutes	Walk 30 minutes	Walk 30 minutes	Walk 30 minutes	Walk 30 minutes	Walk 30 minutes	Walk 30 minutes
Breakfast Slow-cooker oatmeal♥ 3 CholestOff Metamucil	**Breakfast (on the road)** At Au Bon Pain: Oatmeal with raisins, almonds, brown sugar, and fat-free milk Berries 3 CholestOff Metamucil	**Breakfast** Microwave oatmeal♥ 3 CholestOff Metamucil	**Breakfast** Veggie omelet♥ Soy sausages Whole wheat toast Orange sections 3 CholestOff Metamucil	**Breakfast** Cheerios Soy milk Flaxseeds Raisins Walnuts 3 CholestOff Metamucil	**Breakfast** Oatmeal Soy milk Flaxseeds Dried cranberries Orange sections 3 CholestOff Metamucil	**Breakfast** Almond oat pancakes♥ 3 CholestOff Metamucil
Snack Soy nuts	**Snack** Blueberry flax muffin♥ Soy yogurt	**Snack** Soy chips or "nuggets"	**Snack** Blueberry flax muffin♥	**Snack** Apple	**Snack** Soy yogurt Apple	**Snack** Soy latte
Lunch At Burger King: BK veggie burger Side salad with Ken's Light Italian Dressing	**Lunch (brown bag)** Almond nut butter and banana sandwich on 100% whole wheat bread Bag of mini carrots	**Lunch** Vegetarian chili♥ served over brown rice with "baked" tortilla chips	**Lunch** Four-mushroom barley soup♥ Deli club sandwich♥ Baked potato chips	**Lunch** At the Japanese restaurant: Edamame Miso soup Sautéed tofu with vegetables Brown rice	**Lunch** Salsa♥ with "light" tortilla chips Mexican bean wrap♥	**Lunch** Tuna and tofu salad♥

Snack Apple	**Snack** Soy latte	**Snack** Apple	**Snack** Almonds Apple	**Snack** Soy yogurt	**Snack** Veggies/creamy garlic hummus♥	**Snack** Pear
Dinner** 3 CholestOff Metamucil Raspberry walnut salad♥ Grilled tuna steaks♥ Grilled asparagus♥ Black beans♥ served over brown rice Dark chocolate	**Dinner**** 3 CholestOff Metamucil Minestrone soup♥ Edamame dip♥ served with whole wheat pita crisps♥ Pasta with mushroom marinara♥ Sautéed spinach♥ Baked stuffed apples♥	**Dinner**** 3 CholestOff Metamucil Lentil soup♥ Walnut-encrusted salmon♥ Peas with dill♥ Roasted tomatoes with garlic♥ Blueberry dessert smoothie♥	**Dinner**** 3 CholestOff Metamucil Spinach salad with grilled portobello mushrooms♥ Soy chicken patties♥ Mashed potatoes with chickpeas♥ Garlicky broccoli♥ Dark chocolate	**Dinner**** 3 CholestOff Metamucil Eggplant caviar♥ with pita crisps Grilled halibut with Mediterranean salsa♥ Sautéed green beans♥ Wild rice with pecans♥ Dark chocolate	**Dinner**** 3 CholestOff Metamucil At P. F. Chang: Vegetarian lettuce wraps with tofu Miso glazed salmon Korean-style cauliflower Dark chocolate	**Dinner**** 3 CholestOff Metamucil BBQ: Curried okra♥ Grilled veggie burger with the works♥ Baked beans (vegetarian) Corn on the cob Apple pie♥

♥ Heart-healthy recipe included.

* Note portion sizes and daily calorie intake to ensure you are eating 10 percent fewer calories than you typically did.

** Optional glass of red wine with dinner.

Week 2*

Monday	Tuesday	Wednesday	Thursday	Friday	Saturday	Sunday
Walk 30 minutes	Walk 30 minutes	Walk 30 minutes	Walk 30 minutes	Walk 30 minutes	Walk 30 minutes	Walk 30 minutes
Breakfast 3 CholestOff Metamucil Oatmeal/oat bran Soy milk Flaxseeds Dried cranberries Kiwi slices	**Breakfast (at the diner)** 3 CholestOff Metamucil Oatmeal with cinnamon, raisins, and slivered almonds Cantaloupe	**Breakfast** 3 CholestOff Metamucil Oatmeal/oat bran Soy milk Flaxseeds Dried cranberries Fresh strawberries	**Breakfast** 3 CholestOff Metamucil Cheerios/oat bran Soy milk Flaxseeds Raisins	**Breakfast** 3 CholestOff Metamucil Egg white omelet with cheese♥ 100% whole wheat toast Orange sections	**Breakfast** 3 CholestOff Metamucil Oatmeal/oat bran Soy milk Flaxseeds Fresh blueberries	**Breakfast** 3 CholestOff Metamucil Oat-apple-flax pancakes♥ Orange sections
Snack Banana Almonds	**Snack** Soy latte Blueberry flax muffin	**Snack** Kind Pomegranate Blueberry Pistachio Bar	**Snack** Apple	**Snack** Vanilla soy smoothie with flaxseeds♥	**Snack** Almonds Apple rings	**Snack** Almonds
Lunch At Johnny Rockets restaurant: Boca burger with grilled onions, lettuce, tomato, pickle, and mustard	**Lunch** Curried lentil and potato soup♥ Pizza with caramelized onions and roasted tofu♥	**Lunch** Healthy bean quesadilla♥	**Lunch** Walnut hummus and vegetable wrap♥	**Lunch** Chinese takeout: Mixed vegetable stir-fry with tofu	**Lunch** Falafel pita pockets with yogurt sauce♥ Side of butternut squash fries♥	**Lunch** Tuna salad♥

Snack Apple Soy milk-based smoothie	**Snack** Apple Soy crisps	**Snack** Apple	**Snack** Smoky baba ghanoush♥ on whole wheat pita crisps♥	**Snack** Baby carrots	**Snack** Raw veggies with garlicky bean dip♥	**Snack** Pear
Dinner* 3 CholestOff Metamucil Vegetable soup with tofu♥ Grilled grouper with fruit salsa♥ Roasted asparagus♥ Lentil pilaf Green tea Apple and nut sweet treat♥	**Dinner*** 3 CholestOff Metamucil Tropical salad♥ Crusty Italian bread Eggplant lasagna♥ Green tea Dark chocolate	**Dinner*** 3 CholestOff Metamucil Mandarin orange salad♥ Shrimp and tofu vegetable stir fry♥ Brown rice Green tea Dark chocolate	**Dinner*** 3 CholestOff Metamucil At the Japanese restaurant: Green salad with ginger dressing Miso soup Edamame Assorted sashimi Brown rice Green tea Bean brownies♥	**Dinner*** 3 CholestOff Metamucil Spinach salad with apples, pears, and walnuts♥ Chicken with 40 cloves of garlic♥ Barley risotto♥ Okra succotash♥ Green tea Dark chocolate	**Dinner*** 3 CholestOff Metamucil At the steakhouse restaurant: Salad from salad bar with spinach, assorted veggies, chickpeas, and olive oil vinaigrette Grilled salmon Baked potato Steamed broccoli	**Dinner*** 3 CholestOff Metamucil Arugula salad♥ Pasta with meatballs♥ Roasted baby eggplant and tomatoes♥ Crusty Italian bread Chocolate almond decadence with raspberry coulis♥

♥ Heart-healthy recipe included.

* Note portion sizes and daily calorie intake to ensure you are eating 10 percent fewer calories than you typically did.

** Optional glass of red wine with dinner.

Appendix 4

HEART-HEALTHY RECIPES

WEEK ONE

Monday's Recipes

Slow-Cooker Oatmeal

YIELD: 8 SERVINGS

1 cup steel-cut oats (preferably organically grown)

1 cup dried cranberries

2 cups water

4 cups light soy milk

1 ripe banana, sliced

½ cup ground flaxseeds

Pinch of cinnamon

Chopped almonds, optional

Brown sugar, optional

Fat-free half-and-half, optional

Spray inside of a slow cooker insert with nonstick cooking spray. Combine all ingredients in crock pot and stir. Cover and cook on low for 8 to 9 hours. Garnish with chopped almonds, brown sugar, and fat-free half-and-half, if desired.

Nutritional information per serving (⅛ of recipe, 224 grams or approximately 1 cup):

Calories: 195, Fat: 5 g, Cholesterol: 0 mg, Sodium: 52 mg, Carbohydrate: 34 g, Dietary Fiber: 5 g, Sugars: 7 g, Protein: 6 g

Note: Computerized nutrition analyses were performed using arbitrary recipe serving sizes (portions that I typically eat) and not using standardized "serving sizes," as listed under the new Food Pyramid guidelines. In all of the following recipes, whenever possible, I recommend using organically grown fruits, vegetables, grains, and other products; fish that has been caught in the wild; and free-range poultry that has been raised without hormones and antibiotics.

Raspberry Walnut Salad

YIELD: 1 SERVING (WITH DRESSING LEFT OVER)

Dressing:

⅓ cup fresh raspberries

1 tablespoon balsamic vinegar

2 teaspoons Dijon mustard

1 tablespoon water

1 garlic clove, minced

½ teaspoon honey

Salt

Freshly ground black pepper

5 tablespoons extra virgin olive oil

2 tablespoons chopped shallots

In a blender or food processor, combine all dressing ingredients except the oil and shallots and process until smooth. Slowly add the oil and blend until dressing is a thick consistency. Stir in shallots. Chill dressing until salad is served.

Salad:

1 teaspoon extra virgin olive oil

1 teaspoon honey

1 ounce chopped walnuts

2 cups mixed greens (preferably organically grown)

1 teaspoon finely crumbled goat cheese

1 pear, thinly sliced

Preheat oven to 350°F. Spray a baking sheet with nonstick cooking spray. In a small bowl, combine oil and honey. Add walnuts and toss to coat. Spread walnuts on the baking sheet and bake in oven until golden brown, approximately 10 minutes. Place greens in salad bowl; add cheese, walnuts, and pear slices. Add desired amount of salad dressing and toss.

Nutritional information per serving (salad with approximately 1 tablespoon dressing):

Calories: 445, Fat: 31 g, Cholesterol: 5 mg, Sodium: 83 mg, Carbohydrate: 41 g, Dietary Fiber: 9 g, Sugars: 23 g, Protein: 8 g

Grilled Tuna Steaks

YIELD: 2 SERVINGS

2 tuna steaks (6 ounces each)

½ teaspoon salt

¼ teaspoon freshly ground black pepper

¼ cup apricot jam

1 tablespoon Dijon mustard

Lemon wedges, for garnish

Preheat grill (medium-high heat) or broiler. Season tuna steaks with salt and pepper. Combine jam and mustard in a small bowl. Baste fish with half the jam mixture. Place tuna on grill. Cook for 5 minutes, flip, and spread with remaining jam mixture. Grill on the other side until center is slightly pink, about 5 more minutes. Garnish with fresh lemon slices.

Nutritional information per serving (1 tuna steak):

Calories: 343, Fat: 8 g, Cholesterol: 64 mg, Sodium: 760 mg, Carbohydrate: 26 g, Dietary Fiber: 0 g, Sugars: 25 g, Protein: 40 g

Grilled Asparagus

YIELD: 4 SERVINGS

1 pound fresh asparagus

1 tablespoon extra virgin olive oil

1 teaspoon balsamic vinegar

Salt

White pepper

Preheat grill (medium-high heat) or broiler. Trim and discard ends from asparagus by breaking off stalks at the point they are tough. Lightly coat asparagus spears with oil. Grill over high heat for approximately five minutes until done (turn often to prevent charring). Drizzle vinegar over spears and season with salt and white pepper to taste. Serve hot.

Nutritional information per serving (¼ of recipe, 118 grams or approximately 4 ounces):

Calories: 63, Fat: 4 g, Cholesterol: 0 mg, Sodium: 73 mg,
Carbohydrate: 5 g, Dietary Fiber: 2 g, Sugars: 3 g, Protein: 2 g

Black Beans and Rice

YIELD: 4 SERVINGS

1 tablespoon extra virgin olive oil

3 tablespoons chopped red onion

2 garlic cloves, mashed

1 can (15 ounces) black beans, rinsed and drained

½ cup reduced-sodium chicken broth

1 tablespoon balsamic vinegar

¼ teaspoon ground cumin

¼ teaspoon dried oregano

Dash fresh lemon juice

Dash cayenne pepper

2 cups cooked brown rice

In a saucepan, heat olive oil and sauté onion and garlic until onion is wilted, about 5 minutes. Add remaining ingredients except rice and simmer for 15 minutes, stirring occasionally. Serve over ½ cup cooked brown rice.

Nutritional information per serving (¼ of recipe, approximately ½ cup beans and ½ cup cooked brown rice):

Calories: 210, Fat: 4 g, Cholesterol: 0 mg, Sodium: 294 mg,
Carbohydrate: 39 g, Dietary Fiber: 7 g, Sugars: 2 g, Protein: 7 g

Tuesday's Recipes

Blueberry Flax Muffins

YIELD: 12 SERVINGS

¾ cup oat bran

1 cup light soy milk

¼ cup egg substitute (such as Egg Beaters)

¾ cup unsweetened applesauce

¼ cup canola oil

½ cup raisins

1 cup frozen blueberries (unsweetened, slightly thawed)

½ cup sugar

½ cup all-purpose flour

½ cup whole wheat flour

½ cup ground flaxseeds

½ cup brown sugar, packed

1 teaspoon baking soda

¼ teaspoon cinnamon

Preheat oven to 425°F. Spray a 12-cup muffin tin with nonstick cooking spray. Combine first six ingredients in a large mixing bowl. Fold in blueberries, gently stirring until coated. In a separate bowl, mix remaining ingredients. Combine both mixtures and stir until just blended. Fill muffin cups two-thirds full with batter and bake until golden brown, about 20 minutes.

Nutritional information per serving (1 muffin):

Calories: 232, Fat: 7 g, Cholesterol: 0 mg, Sodium: 130 mg, Carbohydrate: 41 g, Dietary Fiber: 4 g, Sugars: 25 g, Protein: 5 g

Minestrone Soup

YIELD: 12 SERVINGS

1 tablespoon extra virgin olive oil

2 medium zucchini, cut into small pieces

3 carrots, cut into small pieces

1 medium onion, chopped

2 garlic cloves, sliced

2 cups kale, chopped, stems removed

1 can (28 ounces) diced tomatoes flavored with basil, garlic, and oregano

2 cups water

1 quart vegetable broth

1 can (15 ounces) cannellini beans, rinsed and drained

½ cup uncooked orzo

¼ teaspoon salt

¼ teaspoon freshly ground black pepper

10 plant-based meatless meatballs

Asiago cheese, grated, optional

Heat oil in a large pot. Add zucchini, carrots, onion, and garlic; sauté over high heat until onion is transparent. Add kale and sauté until wilted. Reduce heat to medium. Add tomatoes, water, broth, and beans. Simmer until carrots are cooked, about 20 minutes. Meanwhile, cook orzo in a separate pot. After 20 minutes, add cooked orzo to soup. Add salt, pepper, and meatballs and simmer a few more minutes until meatballs are hot. Pour into bowls and sprinkle with cheese.

Nutritional information per serving (1⁄12 of recipe, 323 grams or approximately 1½ cups):

Calories: 211, Fat: 5 g, Cholesterol: 0 mg, Sodium: 1,005 mg, Carbohydrate: 25 g, Dietary Fiber: 5 g, Sugars: 5 g, Protein: 17 g

Edamame Dip

YIELD: 8 SERVINGS

2 cups frozen shelled edamame, thawed

1 cup frozen organic spinach, thawed

6 tablespoons extra virgin olive oil

3 tablespoons fresh lemon juice (about 1 lemon)

1 clove garlic

1½ teaspoons salt

¼ teaspoon black pepper

Add the edamame, spinach, olive oil, lemon juice, garlic, salt, and pepper to your food processor. Blend until the mixture is as creamy and smooth as possible, stopping to scrape the sides as needed. If the dip is too thick, add 1 tablespoon of water at a time to reach the desired consistency. Serve the dip with whole wheat pita chips or raw vegetables, or use it as a sandwich spread. Store covered in the refrigerator, or you can freeze it.

Nutritional information per serving (⅛ of recipe):

Calories: 143, Fat: 13 g, Cholesterol: 0 mg, Sodium: 442 mg, Carbohydrate: 5 g, Dietary Fiber: 2 g, Sugars: 1 g, Protein: 4 g

Whole Wheat Pita Crisps

YIELD: 1 SERVING

1 large 100% whole wheat pita bread

Dash paprika

Cut pita into 4 wedges. Place pita on baking sheet and sprinkle with paprika. Toast in toaster oven until crisp.

Nutritional information per serving (1 pita):

Calories: 120, Fat: 1 g, Cholesterol: 0 mg, Sodium: 240 mg, Carbohydrate: 25 g, Dietary Fiber: 3 g, Sugars: 0 g, Protein: 4 g

Pasta with Mushroom Marinara

YIELD: 6 SERVINGS

1 package (16 ounces) 100% whole wheat pasta (I use Gia Russa brand, imported from Italy)

3 tablespoons extra virgin olive oil

2 medium onions, diced

1 teaspoon salt

½ teaspoon freshly ground black pepper

3 garlic cloves, minced

8 ounces button mushrooms, sliced

⅓ cup dry red wine

¾ cup fresh parsley, chopped

½ teaspoon oregano

1 (28-ounce) can crushed tomatoes

1 tablespoon sugar

Fresh basil leaves, thinly sliced, optional

Freshly grated Parmesan cheese, optional

Cook pasta according to package directions; drain and set aside. In a large saucepan, heat olive oil over medium heat. Add onions, ½ teaspoon salt, and ¼ teaspoon pepper and cook, covered, for approximately 8 minutes, stirring occasionally. Add the garlic and mushrooms and cook covered for an additional 8 minutes, stirring occasionally. Add the wine, stir, and cook uncovered for 3 more minutes. Add the parsley, the oregano, and the remaining salt and pepper, stir, and cook uncovered an additional 4 minutes. Add the tomatoes and sugar and cook for 5 more minutes, stirring often. Transfer pasta to plates, spoon the sauce over the top, and garnish with basil and cheese, if desired. Serve immediately.

Nutritional information per serving (approximately 1 cup sauce over 1½ cups cooked pasta):

Calories: 338, Fat: 8 g, Cholesterol: 0 mg, Sodium: 679 mg, Carbohydrate: 61 g, Dietary Fiber: 10 g, Sugars: 11 g, Protein: 11 g

Sautéed Spinach with Garlic

YIELD: 4 SERVINGS

2 tablespoons extra virgin olive oil

4 garlic cloves, minced

2 bags (10 ounces each) washed spinach (preferably organic)

½ cup reduced-sodium chicken broth

Salt and freshly ground black pepper

In a wok or large skillet, heat olive oil over medium heat. Add garlic and sauté until garlic is golden brown. Add spinach and broth, cover, and steam until spinach is just wilted, about 4 minutes. Season to taste with salt and pepper and serve hot.

Nutritional information per serving (¼ of recipe, 182 grams or approximately ¾ cup cooked spinach):

Calories: 102, Fat: 8 g, Cholesterol: 0 mg, Sodium: 327 mg, Carbohydrate: 6 g, Dietary Fiber: 3 g, Sugars: 0 g, Protein: 5 g

Baked Stuffed Apples

YIELD: 6 SERVINGS

6 medium red apples (I use McIntosh)

2 cups water

Juice of ½ lemon (approximately 2 tablespoons)

½ cup pure maple syrup (preferably dark amber grade A)

½ cup raisins

½ cup chopped walnuts

1 teaspoon cinnamon

Preheat oven to 350°F. Core apples and place in water mixed with lemon juice while you prepare the additional ingredients. Mix syrup with raisins, walnuts, and cinnamon. Remove apples from water and fill apples with raisin mixture and place in a baking dish. Pour 1 cup of lemon water in the bottom of the dish. Bake uncovered until tender, about 60 minutes. Drizzle juice from bottom of dish over apples and serve hot.

Nutritional information per serving (1 apple):

Calories: 251, Fat: 7 g, Cholesterol: 0 mg, Sodium: 7 mg, Carbohydrate: 50 g, Dietary Fiber: 5 g, Sugars: 40 g, Protein: 2 g

Wednesday's Recipes

Microwave Oatmeal

YIELD: 1 SERVING

2 packets plain instant oatmeal (I like McCann's "Quick & Easy" steel-cut oatmeal and use about ¼ cup)

1 tablespoon oat bran

2 tablespoons ground flaxseeds

1 cup light soy milk

2 tablespoons real maple syrup or 2 packets Splenda, optional

1 tablespoon dried cranberries or raisins, optional

Fat-free half-and-half, optional

Chopped almonds, optional

Place oatmeal, oat bran, flaxseeds, soy milk, sweetener, and cranberries in a large microwave-safe dish and stir. Microwave on high for 2 minutes (5 minutes if using McCann's oatmeal). Stir; top with fat-free half-and-half and chopped almonds, if desired.

Nutritional information per serving (approximately 1½ cups):
Calories: 391, Fat: 11 g, Cholesterol: 0 mg, Sodium: 261 mg, Carbohydrate: 60 g, Dietary Fiber: 11 g, Sugars: 0 g, Protein: 17 g

Vegetarian Chili

Serve over brown rice accompanied with baked tortilla chips.

YIELD: 10 SERVINGS

2 green bell peppers, chopped

1 cup chopped onion

3 garlic cloves, minced

1 tablespoon extra virgin olive oil

1 can (15 ounces) black beans, rinsed and drained

1 can (15 ounces) kidney beans, rinsed and drained

1 cup chunky salsa (medium or hot, depending on preference)

2 cans (28 ounces each) diced tomatoes

1 cup frozen corn

2 pouches (2 cups) Boca Meatless Ground Burger (found in the frozen foods section of some supermarkets)

1 can (4.5 ounces) chopped green chilies, drained

2 tablespoons chili powder

½ teaspoon cumin

¼ teaspoon cayenne pepper

Soy cheddar cheese, shredded, optional

In a large soup pot, sauté green pepper, onion, and garlic in olive oil over medium-high heat until onion is translucent, about 5 minutes. Add remaining ingredients except for soy cheese and bring to a boil. Reduce heat, cover, and simmer for 30 minutes, stirring occasionally. Garnish with shredded soy cheddar cheese.

Nutritional information per serving (1⁄10 of recipe, 363 grams or approximately 1½ cups chili):

Calories: 186, Fat: 2 g, Cholesterol: 0 mg, Sodium: 854 mg, Carbohydrate: 33 g, Dietary Fiber: 9 g, Sugars: 9 g, Protein: 12 g

Lentil Soup

YIELD: 12 SERVINGS

1 pound French green lentils

2 teaspoons sea salt

⅓ cup extra virgin olive oil

1 bay leaf

2 stalks celery, chopped

1 cup chopped onion

2 carrots, chopped

4 garlic cloves, mashed

2 cups chopped kale, stems removed

1 carton (26 ounces) Parmalat "Pomi" chopped tomatoes (imported from Italy without added sodium)

3 cans (14 ounces each) reduced-sodium chicken broth

¼ teaspoon freshly ground black pepper

Fresh parsley, for garnish

Freshly grated Parmesan cheese, for garnish

Additional extra virgin olive oil, for garnish

Wash lentils and place in a large soup pot. Cover lentils with water and add 1 teaspoon sea salt. Bring to a boil and cook for 5 minutes. Drain and rinse lentils and set aside. Heat olive oil in soup pot with bay leaf over medium heat. Add celery, onions, carrots, and garlic and cook for five minutes, stirring occasionally. Add kale and cook until wilted, approximately 5 minutes, then stir in tomatoes. Add chicken broth, remaining salt, and lentils to pot. Stir all ingredients and bring to a boil over high heat. Reduce heat and simmer uncovered for 15 minutes. Add pepper and remove bay leaf before serving. Divide into bowls and garnish with parsley, freshly grated Parmesan cheese, and a touch of extra virgin olive oil, if desired.

Nutritional information per serving (1⁄12 of recipe, 258 grams or approximately 1¼ cups soup):

Calories: 220, Fat: 6 g, Cholesterol: 0 mg, Sodium: 742 mg, Carbohydrate: 30 g, Dietary Fiber: 7 g, Sugars: 5 g, Protein: 12 g

Walnut-Encrusted Salmon

YIELD: 4 SERVINGS (SERVING SIZE: 1 SALMON FILLET)

3 garlic cloves

¾ cup walnuts

½ cup cilantro

2 tablespoons extra virgin olive oil

4 salmon fillets, preferably wild, about 6 ounces each

1 teaspoon kosher salt

¼ teaspoon freshly ground black pepper

Fresh lemon slices, for garnish

Preheat oven to 450°F. Mince the garlic in a food processor. Add the walnuts and process until walnuts are finely chopped. Add cilantro and process until mixture is thick and pasty. Drizzle in olive oil and process until blended. Place salmon on a foil-lined baking tray. Season both sides with salt and pepper. Spread the walnut mixture evenly over the fish. Bake salmon for 20 minutes or until fish flakes easily with a fork. Garnish with fresh lemon slices.

Nutritional information per serving (1 salmon fillet):

Calories: 456, Fat: 32 g, Cholesterol: 94 mg, Sodium: 658 mg, Carbohydrate: 4 g, Dietary Fiber: 2 g, Sugars: 0 g, Protein: 37 g

Peas with Dill

YIELD: 6 SERVINGS

2 tablespoons extra virgin olive oil

1 large onion, chopped

2 packages (10 ounces each) frozen sweet peas

½ cup fresh dill, chopped

3 medium red potatoes

¾ cup water

Salt

Freshly ground pepper

Lemon wedges, for garnish

Heat oil in large frying pan and sauté onion over medium heat until translucent. Add peas and dill. Quarter potatoes and add to pan. Add water, cover pan, and simmer until potato is soft but not overdone, stirring occasionally. Add salt and pepper to taste. Serve warm. Garnish with fresh lemon wedges.

Nutritional information per serving (⅙ of recipe, 241 grams or approximately 1 cup):

Calories: 190, Fat: 5 g, Cholesterol: 0 mg, Sodium: 258 mg, Carbohydrate: 31 g, Dietary Fiber: 6 g, Sugars: 9 g, Protein: 6 g

Roasted Tomatoes with Garlic

YIELD: 8 SERVINGS

2 pounds plum tomatoes, preferably organic

4 garlic cloves, cut lengthwise into slivers

1 teaspoon salt

½ teaspoon freshly ground black pepper

2 tablespoons extra virgin olive oil

Drizzle of balsamic reduction glaze (I use a commercially prepared brand, Gia Russa from Italy)

½ cup chopped fresh basil, for garnish

Put oven rack in center position and preheat oven to 450°F. Cut tomatoes in half crosswise. Arrange tomatoes with cut side up in a lightly oiled shallow baking pan. Stud the tomato halves with slivers of garlic, then sprinkle with salt and pepper. Drizzle tomatoes evenly with olive oil and balsamic reduction glaze. Roast until soft, about 20 minutes. Remove from oven and serve warm. Garnish with fresh basil.

Nutritional information per serving (⅛ of recipe, 135 grams or approximately ½ cup):

Calories: 78, Fat: 4 g, Cholesterol: 0 mg, Sodium: 304 mg, Carbohydrate: 11 g, Dietary Fiber: 2 g, Sugars: 4 g, Protein: 2 g

Blueberry Dessert Smoothie

YIELD: 2 SERVINGS (SERVING SIZE: APPROXIMATELY 2 CUPS)

1 cup vanilla soy milk

2 tablespoons Nesquik chocolate powder

1 cup frozen blueberries, unsweetened

1 cup frozen sliced peaches, unsweetened

In a blender, combine all ingredients and blend to desired consistency. Pour into glasses and serve.

Nutritional information per serving (approximately 14 fluid ounces):

Calories: 149, Fat: 2 g, Cholesterol: 2 mg, Sodium: 102 mg, Carbohydrate: 29 g, Dietary Fiber: 4 g, Sugars: 18 g, Protein: 16 g

Thursday's Recipes

Veggie Omelet

YIELD: 1 SERVING

¼ cup asparagus, chopped

1 tablespoon water

2 teaspoons canola oil

¼ cup jarred sweet red peppers (found in the condiments section of most supermarkets)

½ medium Vidalia onion, chopped

6 egg whites

1 ounce soy cheddar cheese, shredded

Salt

Freshly ground pepper

Trim and discard ends from asparagus by breaking off stalks at the point they are tough. Chop the tender portions of the spears into small pieces. Microwave in microwave-safe bowl with water until soft, about 2 minutes. Heat oil in frying pan. Add vegetables and sauté over medium-high heat until cooked (onion is transparent). Whisk egg whites together until a froth forms. Add egg whites and fry until omelet has reached desired consistency. Top with shredded cheese, cover, and continue heating until cheese has just melted. Season to taste with salt and pepper, if desired, and serve warm.

Nutritional information per serving (1 omelet):

Calories: 261, Fat: 13 g, Cholesterol: 0 mg, Sodium: 840 mg, Carbohydrate: 8 g, Dietary Fiber: 2 g, Sugars: 2 g, Protein: 29 g

Four-Mushroom Barley Soup

YIELD: 10 SERVINGS

9 cups reduced-sodium chicken broth

½ ounce dried porcini mushrooms

½ ounce dried shiitake mushrooms

¼ cup canola oil

1 large onion, chopped

2 medium shallots, finely chopped

8-ounce package baby bella or cremini mushrooms, stemmed, cleaned, and diced

12-ounce package white button mushrooms, stemmed, cleaned, and quartered

1 teaspoon kosher salt

2 carrots, peeled and chopped into small pieces

3 garlic cloves, minced

1 cup whole-grain barley

1 bay leaf

¼ teaspoon dried thyme

Shredded soy or regular part-skim mozzarella cheese, optional

Heat 1½ cups chicken broth. Add porcini and shiitake mushrooms to broth and soak, covered, until soft, about 30 minutes. Remove mushrooms from broth and chop into small pieces; set aside. Strain soaking liquid and set aside. Heat the oil in a large stockpot over medium heat. Add onions and shallots and cook until onions are translucent, about 5 minutes. Add the baby bella and button mushrooms and salt. Cook, stirring frequently, until mushrooms are tender, about 10 minutes. Add carrots and garlic, stir, and cook an additional minute. Add remaining chicken broth, porcini and shiitake soaking liquid, porcini and shiitake mushrooms, barley, bay leaf, and thyme. Bring to a boil, stir, and cover; reduce heat and simmer about 1 hour. Remove and discard bay leaf before serving. Sprinkle with shredded mozzarella cheese before serving, if desired.

Nutritional information per serving (⅒ of recipe, 351 grams or approximately 1½ cups soup):

Calories: 157, Fat: 6 g, Cholesterol: 0 mg, Sodium: 744 mg, Carbohydrate: 20 g, Dietary Fiber: 5 g, Sugars: 2 g, Protein: 7 g

Deli Club Sandwich

YIELD: 1 SERVING

2 slices 100% whole wheat bread

4 slices Smart Deli roast-turkey-style soy deli slices

1 ounce light cheddar cheese

½ avocado, peeled and sliced

¼ cup chopped spinach

2 slices tomato

1 slice red onion

Mustard

Toast whole wheat bread. Combine all ingredients into sandwich and add condiments to taste.

Nutritional information per serving (1 sandwich):

Calories: 353, Fat: 10 g, Cholesterol: 0 mg, Sodium: 1134 mg, Carbohydrate: 40 g, Dietary Fiber: 10 g, Sugars: 14 g, Protein: 29 g

Spinach Salad with Grilled Portobello Mushrooms

YIELD: 2 SERVINGS

4 cups washed spinach leaves, preferably organically grown

2 large ripe tomatoes, diced

2 large portobello mushrooms

2 tablespoons extra virgin olive oil

3 garlic cloves, minced

Juice of ½ fresh lemon

Salt

Freshly ground black pepper

Balsamic glaze

Heat grill to medium-high heat. Chop spinach into small pieces and divide spinach between two salad plates. Top each with chopped tomatoes. Wash and dry mushrooms, removing stems. In a small pot, heat olive oil and sauté garlic with lemon juice, salt, and pepper until garlic is browned. Brush mushroom caps (both sides) generously with olive oil mixture. Grill mushrooms over medium heat, stem side down, about 8 minutes. Turn and grill tops for 6 to 8 minutes more. The mushrooms should be browned and tender. Remove from grill, cut into quarters, and arrange over spinach salad. Add seasoning to taste. Drizzle salad with balsamic glaze and serve.

Nutritional information per serving (½ of recipe):

Calories: 220, Fat: 15 g, Cholesterol: 0 mg, Sodium: 236 mg, Carbohydrate: 21 g, Dietary Fiber: 5 g, Sugars: 7 g, Protein: 5 g

Soy Chicken Patties

YIELD: 1 SERVING

2 frozen soy-based chicken patties (such as Morningstar Farms), defrosted

1 tablespoon fresh lemon juice

1 teaspoon dried dill

Commercial gravy, optional

Preheat broiler. Line a baking pan with aluminum foil. Place chicken patties on foil, drizzle with lemon juice, and sprinkle with dill. Broil each side until no longer pink, about 2 minutes. Serve with commercial gravy, if desired.

Nutritional information per serving (2 patties):

Calories: 308, Fat: 13 g, Cholesterol: 1 mg, Sodium: 1028 mg, Carbohydrate: 19 g, Dietary Fiber: 7 g, Sugars: 5 g, Protein: 19 g

Mashed Potatoes with Chickpeas

YIELD: 6 SERVINGS

2 pounds baking potatoes, peeled and cut into chunks

1 can (15.5 ounces) chickpeas, rinsed and drained

1 cup light soy milk

½ cup reduced-sodium chicken broth

¼ cup Benecol Light Spread

1 teaspoon salt

½ teaspoon pepper

Commercial gravy, optional

Place potatoes in large saucepan, cover with water, and bring to a boil. Reduce heat and simmer until tender, about 15 minutes. Drain and return potatoes to pan. Add chickpeas and mash using a potato masher. Add soy milk, chicken broth, Benecol, salt and pepper, and stir. Cook an additional 2 minutes, stirring constantly. Serve warm. Top with commercial gravy, if desired.

Nutritional information per serving (⅙ of recipe, 293 grams or approximately 1 cup):

Calories: 255, Fat: 5 g, Cholesterol: 0 mg, Sodium: 751 mg, Carbohydrate: 46 g, Dietary Fiber: 5 g, Sugars: 3 g, Protein: 7 g

Garlicky Broccoli

YIELD: 2 SERVINGS

2 cups broccoli florets

2 tablespoons water

1 tablespoon extra virgin olive oil

2 garlic cloves, minced

1 teaspoon fresh lemon juice

Salt

Freshly ground black pepper

Fresh parsley, for garnish, optional

Place broccoli in a microwave-safe bowl, add water, and cook in microwave on high until tender, about 5 minutes (I like it very well done, about 10 minutes). In a saucepan, combine olive oil, garlic, and lemon juice and cook over low heat for approximately 3 minutes, stirring occasionally, until garlic is golden brown. Pour garlic sauce over drained broccoli, toss, add salt and pepper to taste, and serve. Garnish with fresh parsley, if desired.

Nutritional information per serving (½ of recipe):

Calories: 88, Fat: 7 g, Cholesterol: 0 mg, Sodium: 20 mg, Carbohydrate: 5 g, Dietary Fiber: 2 g, Sugars: 0 g, Protein: 2 g

Friday's Recipes

Eggplant Caviar

YIELD: 12 SERVINGS

3 large eggplants

3 garlic cloves, minced

1 large onion, chopped

4 tablespoons vinegar (I like it with seasoned rice vinegar)

Juice of ½ lemon

2 tablespoons extra virgin olive oil

½ teaspoon salt

Freshly ground black pepper

Preheat oven to 400°F. Roast eggplants, turning frequently, over a grill or in the oven until the skin is charred all over, about 60 minutes. When cool enough, remove stem and skin and place in food processor. Process until pureed. Pour eggplant puree into a large mixing bowl. Add onions, garlic, vinegar, lemon juice, olive oil, salt, and pepper. Mix together and refrigerate for a minimum of 2 hours to allow the dish to chill completely and the flavors to meld.

Nutritional information per serving (1⁄12 of recipe, 138 grams or approximately ½ cup):

Calories: 60, Fat: 3 g, Cholesterol: 0 mg, Sodium: 199 mg, Carbohydrate: 9 g, Dietary Fiber: 1 g, Sugars: 2 g, Protein: 1 g

Grilled Halibut with Mediterranean Salsa

YIELD: 4 SERVINGS

SALSA:

1 pound plum tomatoes, chopped

1 cup chopped arugula

1 large shallot, finely chopped

¼ cup extra virgin olive oil

Juice of 1 lemon

1 can (15 ounces) Great Northern beans, rinsed and drained

1 small jar capers (approximately 3 ounces), drained

¼ teaspoon salt

¼ teaspoon freshly ground black pepper

FISH:

4 halibut steaks (6 ounces each)

2 tablespoons extra virgin olive oil

Salt

Freshly ground black pepper

Lemon slices, for garnish

Combine all the salsa ingredients together in a bowl and mix. Refrigerate for at least one hour. Brush both sides of fish with olive oil and sprinkle with salt and pepper. Grill over medium-high heat for 4 minutes per side or until fish flakes easily. Serve topped with salsa and garnished with fresh lemon slices.

Nutritional information per serving (1 halibut steak plus approximately ¾ cup salsa):

Calories: 412, Fat: 11 g, Cholesterol: 54 mg, Sodium: 692 mg, Carbohydrate: 16 g, Dietary Fiber: 5 g, Sugars: 3 g, Protein: 40 g

Sautéed Green Beans

YIELD: 2 SERVINGS

¾ pound fresh green beans, trimmed

1 tablespoon extra virgin olive oil

2 teaspoons Dijon or stone-ground mustard

Salt

Freshly ground black pepper

Cook beans in a large pot of boiling water until tender-crisp, approximately 3 to 4 minutes. Drain beans and transfer to a bowl of ice water to stop cooking. Drain well and pat dry. Heat oil in a large skillet over medium-high heat. Sauté green beans with mustard and salt and pepper to taste, stirring until heated, about 4 minutes. Serve hot.

Nutritional information per serving (½ of recipe):

Calories: 114, Fat: 7 g, Cholesterol: 0 mg, Sodium: 65 mg, Carbohydrate: 10 g, Dietary Fiber: 6 g, Sugars: 4 g, Protein: 2 g

Wild Rice with Pecans

YIELD: 8 SERVINGS

1 cup wild rice, uncooked

5 cups reduced-sodium chicken broth

1 cup pecan halves

1 cup golden raisins

¼ cup chopped fresh mint

Zest of 1 large orange

½ cup thinly sliced green onions

¼ cup extra virgin olive oil

⅓ cup orange juice

¾ teaspoon salt

½ teaspoon freshly ground black pepper

Rinse rice thoroughly. Place rice in a medium saucepan and add chicken broth. Bring to a rapid boil, then turn heat down and simmer uncovered for 45 minutes. Stir occasionally and check to make sure rice is not too soft. Drain rice and transfer to a large bowl. Add remaining ingredients and toss gently. Refrigerate for one hour, then let stand and serve at room temperature.

Nutritional information per serving (⅛ of recipe, 229 grams or approximately 1 cup):

Calories: 311, Fat: 17 g, Cholesterol: 0 mg, Sodium: 572 mg, Carbohydrate: 35 g, Dietary Fiber: 4 g, Sugars: 17 g, Protein: 7 g

Saturday's Recipes

Salsa

Serve with baked tortilla chips.

YIELD: 8 SERVINGS

½ teaspoon fresh lemon juice

Juice of 1 lime

¼ teaspoon salt

1 pound ripe plum tomatoes, cored and chopped

½ medium Vidalia onion, diced

2 garlic cloves, minced

1 tablespoon jalapeño pepper, chopped

1 teaspoon chopped cilantro

Mix lemon juice, lime juice, and salt in a mixing bowl until salt dissolves. Add tomatoes to juice and stir. Add onions, garlic, jalapeño, and cilantro. Mix together and refrigerate for a minimum of 2 hours to allow the dish to chill completely and the flavors to meld.

Nutritional information per serving (⅛ of recipe, 87 grams or approximately ⅓ cup):

Calories: 22, Fat: 0 g, Cholesterol: 0 mg, Sodium: 76 mg, Carbohydrate: 5 g, Dietary Fiber: 1 g, Sugars: 2 g, Protein: 1 g

Mexican-Inspired Bean Wrap

YIELD: 1 SERVING

1 whole wheat flour tortilla

2 tablespoons guacamole

½ cup canned kidney beans, drained and rinsed

¼ cup spinach leaves

1 cup jarred sweet red peppers (found in condiments section of some supermarkets)

Spread tortilla with guacamole. Add beans, spinach, and peppers. Roll up tortilla and cut in half.

Nutritional information per serving (1 wrap):

Calories: 340, Fat: 6 g, Cholesterol: 0 mg, Sodium: 442 mg, Carbohydrate: 55 g, Dietary Fiber: 10 g, Sugars: 3 g, Protein: 14 g

Creamy Garlic Hummus

Serve with warm whole wheat pita bread.

YIELD: 18 SERVINGS

¾ cup water

½ cup tahini (sesame seed paste, available at health food stores and some supermarkets)

4 large garlic cloves, crushed

2 cans (15.5 ounces each) chickpeas, rinsed and drained

Juice of 1 lemon

¾ teaspoon ground cumin

½ teaspoon salt

¼ teaspoon freshly ground black pepper

1 tablespoon extra virgin olive oil

Fresh parsley, for garnish

Dash paprika, for garnish

Combine the first four ingredients in a food processor and process until smooth. Add lemon juice, cumin, salt, and pepper and process; with motor running, slowly drizzle in the olive oil until smooth. Garnish with parsley and sprinkle with paprika.

Nutritional information per serving (1⁄18 of recipe, 67 grams or approximately ¼ cup):

Calories: 90, Fat: 5 g, Cholesterol: 0 mg, Sodium: 210 mg, Carbohydrate: 9 g, Dietary Fiber: 2 g, Sugars: 0 g, Protein: 3 g

Sunday's Recipes

Almond Oat Pancakes

Serve warm with Benecol Light Spread, sprinkled with powdered sugar and warm Vermont maple syrup, for a real Sunday morning treat.

YIELD: 6 SERVINGS

½ cup almonds, slivered
1¼ cups all-purpose flour
¾ cup old-fashioned oatmeal
3 tablespoons sugar
½ cup ground flaxseeds
1½ teaspoons baking powder
½ teaspoon salt
1½ cups light soy milk
2 tablespoons canola oil
4 egg whites
½ teaspoon almond extract
½ teaspoon white wine vinegar
Additional canola oil for greasing pan
Powdered sugar, optional
Benecol Light Spread, optional
Maple syrup, optional

Heat oven to 350°F. Place almonds in a single layer on a baking sheet lined with aluminum foil. Bake in oven for about 10 minutes, shaking pan periodically to heat evenly. Combine next 6 ingredients in a large nonreactive mixing bowl. In a separate nonreactive bowl, whisk together next 5 ingredients. Combine wet and dry ingredients and whisk until just mixed. Fold in toasted almonds. Coat a large frying pan with canola oil and heat over medium heat. Pour in ¼ cup batter for each pancake. Cook until batter bubbles, then flip with a spatula and cook until bottom is golden. Sprinkle with powdered sugar and top with Benecol and syrup to taste.

Nutritional information per serving (⅙ of batter, 152 grams or approximately ¾ cup batter) (3 pancakes)

Calories: 362, Fat: 16 g, Cholesterol: 0 mg, Sodium: 359 mg, Carbohydrate: 44 g, Dietary Fiber: 7 g, Sugars: 8 g, Protein: 12 g

Tuna and Tofu Salad

YIELD: 2 SERVINGS

Dressing:

1 garlic clove, minced

1 tablespoon balsamic vinegar

1½ teaspoons Dijon mustard

⅛ teaspoon salt

⅛ teaspoon freshly ground black pepper

⅓ cup extra virgin olive oil

Whisk together all dressing ingredients except the oil. Slowly add the oil and mix until dressing is a thick consistency. Chill dressing until dish is served.

Salad:

YIELD: 2 SERVINGS

4 cups red leaf lettuce, washed, dried, and torn

1 large ripe tomato, diced

½ large Vidalia onion, sliced

¼ cup sliced green onions

½ cup sliced button mushrooms

1 block (14-ounce package) extra-firm tofu

12-ounce can water-packed tuna, drained

Arrange lettuce on a large salad plate. Cut tofu into 1-inch cubes and add to salad. Mix tomato and onion and sprinkle over tofu. Top tomato mixture with tuna, then add green onions. Pour chilled dressing over salad before serving.

Nutritional information per serving (½ of recipe):

Calories: 461, Fat: 17 g, Cholesterol: 51 mg, Sodium: 779 mg, Carbohydrate: 15 g, Dietary Fiber: 2 g, Sugars: 7 g, Protein: 60 g

Curried Okra

YIELD: 6 SERVINGS

1 medium onion, chopped

1 tablespoon fresh ginger, peeled and finely chopped

2 cloves garlic, finely chopped

2 tablespoons canola oil

2 teaspoons curry powder

1 can (15.5 ounces) chickpeas, drained and rinsed

1 can (15.5 ounces) whole tomatoes

⅔ cup water

2 packages (10 ounces each) frozen cut okra, unthawed

¾ teaspoon salt

¼ teaspoon freshly ground black pepper

In a large skillet, sauté onion, ginger, and garlic in canola oil over moderately high heat for 2 to 3 minutes. Add curry powder and stir. Add chickpeas, tomatoes, and water, cut tomatoes into small pieces, releasing juices, and bring to a boil. Simmer uncovered, stirring occasionally, for 3 minutes. Add okra, salt, and pepper and simmer, covered, for approximately 10 minutes until okra is tender. Serve warm.

Nutritional information per serving (⅙ of recipe, 288 grams or approximately 1¼ cups):

Calories: 154, Fat: 6 g, Cholesterol: 0 mg, Sodium: 803 mg, Carbohydrate: 21 g, Dietary Fiber: 7 g, Sugars: 6 g, Protein: 6 g

Grilled Veggie Burger with the Works

YIELD: 1 SERVING

1 Morningstar Farms Grillers Prime Veggie Burger

1 whole wheat hamburger bun (or whole wheat English muffin), toasted

½ cup spinach leaves

2 slices tomato

Grilled onions, garlic, and mushrooms, optional

Condiments (ketchup, mustard, relish, jarred sweet red peppers)

Preheat grill. Grill burger according to package directions. Top burger with spinach and tomatoes; add grilled onions, garlic, and mushrooms and condiments as desired.

Nutritional information per serving (1 burger with the works):

Calories: 317, Fat: 11 g, Cholesterol: 1 mg, Sodium: 594 mg, Carbohydrate: 35 g, Dietary Fiber: 8 g, Sugars: 8 g, Protein: 23 g

Apple Pie with Oatmeal Crust

Serve warm with low-fat vanilla ice cream or frozen yogurt and fat-free whipped topping.

YIELD: 8 SERVINGS

CRUST:

⅓ cup old-fashioned oats

2 tablespoons sugar

1¼ cups all-purpose flour

⅛ teaspoon salt

½ cup Benecol Light Spread

¼ cup ice water

FILLING:

2 pounds baking apples (about 5 medium Rome apples), cored, unpeeled, and thinly sliced

Juice of 1 lemon

¼ cup sugar

¼ cup packed dark brown sugar

1 tablespoon all-purpose flour

1 teaspoon grated lemon peel

¼ teaspoon cinnamon

½ teaspoon nutmeg

1 cup raisins

2 teaspoons egg substitute (such as Egg Beaters)

1 tablespoon sugar

Mix oats and sugar in a food processor until finely ground. Mix in flour and salt and process until blended. Add Benecol and pulse until mixture is coarse. Mix in ice water slowly until a dough forms. Remove dough from food processor and divide into two balls of equal size. Place in plastic wrap and chill for one hour. Place one dough ball between two sheets of floured wax paper. Roll dough into 12-inch circle. Repeat with other dough ball. Chill dough until ready to use.

Preheat oven to 450°F. Combine apples and lemon juice in a large mixing bowl and toss to coat. In a separate large bowl, combine sugar, brown sugar, flour, lemon peel, cinnamon, and nutmeg. Mix well. Sprinkle over apple mixture and toss well to coat apples. Add raisins and mix. Place pie crust in pie pan sprayed with nonstick cooking spray. Spray bottom crust with nonstick cooking spray. Spoon apple filling into bottom pie crust. Cover apple pie filling with second pie crust, press edges of dough together, and flute. Cut six slits in pastry top with a sharp knife. Brush top crust lightly with egg substitute and sprinkle with sugar. Place pie on baking sheet and bake at 450°F for 15 minutes. Reduce heat to 375°F and bake until crust is golden brown, about 40 minutes. Cool on wire rack.

Nutritional information per serving (⅛ of recipe, 1 slice of pie):

Calories: 331, Fat: 7 g, Cholesterol: 0 mg, Sodium: 156 mg, Carbohydrate: 67 g, Dietary Fiber: 5 g, Sugars: 45 g, Protein: 3 g

WEEK TWO

Monday's Recipes

Vegetable Soup with Tofu

YIELD: 8 SERVINGS

2 tablespoons canola oil

1 cup chopped zucchini

1 cup chopped onion

1 cup chopped carrots

4 garlic cloves, chopped into small pieces

1 can (28 ounces) whole tomatoes, organic, undrained and coarsely chopped

2 cartons (32 fluid ounces) organic chicken soup broth

1 bag (5 ounces) organic spinach leaves

1 package (14 ounces) organic, super-firm tofu, drained and cubed

Freshly ground black pepper

Freshly shredded Parmesan cheese

Heat canola oil in a large saucepan over medium-high heat. Add zucchini, onion, carrots, and garlic. Sauté until onion has turned a golden brown, stirring vegetables frequently. Add tomatoes and chicken broth and stir. Bring to a boil, then reduce heat to low. Simmer uncovered for 15 minutes. Add spinach and tofu and cook for an additional 5 minutes. Season to taste and top each serving with 1 tablespoon Parmesan cheese, if desired.

Nutritional information per serving (⅛ of recipe, 329 grams or approximately 1½ cups soup topped with 1 tablespoon shredded Parmesan cheese):

Calories: 134, Fat: 7 g, Cholesterol: 6 mg, Sodium: 525 mg, Carbohydrate: 12 g, Dietary Fiber: 3 g, Sugars: 5 g, Protein: 7 g

Grilled Grouper with Fruit Salsa

YIELD: 4 SERVINGS

2 ripe mangoes, peeled, pitted, and diced

2 cups of red seedless grapes, halved

½ cup red onion, chopped

1 tablespoon fresh cilantro, chopped

Juice of ½ lime

½ medium-sized jalapeño pepper, seeded and minced

¼ teaspoon salt

20 ounces of fresh grouper or a similar mild-tasting, white-fleshed fish

2 tablespoons extra virgin olive oil

½ teaspoon salt

½ teaspoon pepper

Lemon wedges, for garnish

Salsa:
In a large mixing bowl, combine the mangoes, grapes, onion, cilantro, lime juice, jalapeño pepper, and salt and mix well. Cover with plastic wrap and chill until fish is served.

Grouper:
Preheat grill to high heat. Rinse grouper and pat dry. Pour a small amount of olive oil on both sides of the fillets and coat lightly. Sprinkle both sides with salt and pepper to taste. Grill grouper approximately 5 minutes per side until fish is no longer pink on the inside and flakes easily with a fork.

Serve grouper immediately, topped with salsa over each fillet. Garnish with fresh lemon wedges.

Nutritional information per serving (1 grouper fillet with ¼ of salsa recipe or approximately 1 cup salsa):

Calories: 329, Fat: 9 g, Cholesterol: 52 mg, Sodium: 514 mg, Carbohydrate: 34 g, Dietary Fiber: 3 g, Sugars: 15 g, Protein: 29 g

Roasted Asparagus with Garlic

YIELD: 4 SERVINGS

1 pound fresh asparagus

1 tablespoon extra virgin olive oil

2 garlic cloves, minced

Salt

Freshly ground black pepper

Juice from ½ fresh lemon

Preheat oven to 500°F. Trim and discard ends from asparagus by breaking off stalks at the point they are tough. Place olive oil and garlic in a large roasting pan. Add asparagus and turn to coat. Add desired amount of salt and pepper and roast uncovered for 10 to 12 minutes. Remove from oven and sprinkle with lemon juice. Serve hot.

Nutritional information per serving (¼ of recipe, 125 grams or approximately 4 ounces):

Calories: 66, Fat: 4 g, Cholesterol: 0 mg, Sodium: 291 mg, Carbohydrate: 6 g, Dietary Fiber: 3 g, Sugars: 3 g, Protein: 3 g

Apple and Nut Sweet Treat

YIELD: 12 SERVINGS

2 Red Delicious apples, cored and cut into chunks

1½ cups coarsely chopped walnuts

1 tablespoon lemon rind, grated

1½ teaspoons cinnamon

2 tablespoons sugar

3 tablespoons red table wine

In a food processor, pulse apples until chopped into small bits. In a mixing bowl, add apples, walnuts, lemon rind, cinnamon, sugar, and wine and blend by hand until all ingredients are well combined. Chill until dish is served.

Nutritional information per serving (1⁄12 of recipe, 57 grams or approximately ¼ cup):

Calories: 128, Fat: 10 g, Cholesterol: 0 mg, Sodium: 1 mg, Carbohydrate: 9 g, Dietary Fiber: 2 g, Sugars: 6 g, Protein: 2 g

Tuesday's Recipes

Curried Lentil and Potato Soup

YIELD: 8 SERVINGS

1 tablespoon extra virgin olive oil

1 cup chopped onions

3 large garlic cloves, minced

2 large carrots, peeled and chopped

1 tablespoon curry powder

2 bay leaves

1 carton (32 ounces) organic reduced-sodium chicken broth

1 can (28 ounces) organic whole tomatoes

2 sun-dried string figs, cut into small pieces, stems removed

1 cup green lentils, sorted and rinsed

2 cups diced red potatoes

½ teaspoon salt

¼ teaspoon pepper

Heat oil over medium heat in a large soup pot. Add onions, garlic, and carrots and sauté for approximately 10 minutes until onions are softened and beginning to caramelize. Add curry and bay leaves and stir to coat onions. Add chicken broth, tomatoes, figs, and lentils, stirring often to break up tomatoes. Bring to a boil, reduce heat, and simmer for 30 minutes, stirring occasionally. Add potatoes, increase heat to medium, and cook uncovered for an additional 30 minutes until potatoes are soft. Remove from heat, discard bay leaves, and place two-thirds of lentil mixture in a food processor. Add salt and pepper and process until mixture has pureed. Add puree back into soup pot, stir, and serve warm.

Nutritional information per serving (⅛ of recipe, 328 grams or approximately 1½ cups soup):

Calories: 187, Fat: 2 g, Cholesterol: 3 mg, Sodium: 633 mg, Carbohydrate: 33 g, Dietary Fiber: 7 g, Sugars: 8 g, Protein: 8 g

Pizza with Caramelized Onions and Roasted Tofu

This easy-to-make and highly nutritious pizza is loaded with taste and lacks only the gobs of saturated fat contained in regular pizza. Who knew whole wheat pizza could taste this good?

YIELD: 8 SERVINGS

3 tablespoons extra virgin olive oil

2 tablespoons balsamic vinegar

¼ teaspoon salt

¼ teaspoon black pepper

1 large red onion, thinly sliced

7 ounces of firm, cubed tofu (½ a typical package), drained

1 tablespoon extra virgin olive oil

3 large garlic cloves, sliced

1 large Boboli 100% whole wheat pizza crust

2 teaspoons olive oil

1 packet Boboli pizza sauce

6 large black olives, pitted and sliced

Toppings:

Preheat oven to high broil. In a large mixing bowl, mix olive oil and balsamic vinegar, salt, and pepper. Line a baking sheet with aluminum foil and spray with olive oil cooking spray. Place onions on baking sheet and baste with balsamic mixture until onions are well coated. Add tofu to balsamic mixture, turn to coat, and set aside. Broil onions for approximately 6 minutes, turning occasionally, until tender and browned. Remove from oven and set aside, reduce heat in oven to 450°F. In a small skillet, add olive oil and garlic and sauté until garlic is browned. Remove from heat and set aside.

Pizza:

Baste Boboli pizza crust with 2 teaspoons olive oil. Add packet of tomato sauce and spread evenly. Top sauce with onions, garlic, tofu (discard marinade), and olives. Bake pizza on oven rack or pizza stone for 10 minutes. Serve immediately.

Nutritional information per serving (⅛ of pizza):

Calories: 209, Fat: 12 g, Cholesterol: 0 mg, Sodium: 320 mg, Carbohydrate: 20 g, Dietary Fiber: 3 g, Sugars: 3 g, Protein: 7 g

Tropical Salad

Dressing:

2 garlic cloves

1 tablespoon reduced-fat mayonnaise

1 tablespoon Dijon mustard

2 tablespoons water

¼ teaspoon white pepper

¼ cup balsamic vinegar

1 teaspoon honey

¾ cup canola oil

Mix all ingredients except canola oil in a food processor, slowly drizzle in oil, blending until smooth.

Salad:

YIELD: 4 SERVINGS

1 cup baby spinach

2 cups mixed greens

1 ripe avocado, sliced

1 mango, cut into small chunks

1 cup sliced strawberries

½ cup toasted walnuts

2 tablespoons crumbled goat cheese

Place greens in salad bowl; add avocado, mango, and strawberries. Place walnuts on a sheet of aluminum foil and toast for 3 minutes or until slightly browned. Add walnuts and cheese to salad. Add desired amount of salad dressing and toss.

Nutritional information per serving (¼ of salad recipe with approximately 1 tablespoon of dressing):

Calories: 339, Fat: 28 g, Cholesterol: 6 mg, Sodium: 74 mg, Carbohydrate: 20 g, Dietary Fiber: 7 g, Sugars: 5 g, Protein: 6 g

Eggplant Lasagna

YIELD: 8 SERVINGS

2 medium eggplants

1 teaspoon salt

2 tablespoons extra virgin olive oil

8 ounces sliced white mushrooms

4 garlic cloves, minced

1 can (28 ounces) organic whole peeled tomatoes, undrained, coarsely chopped

2 tablespoons canned organic tomato paste

2 large ripe tomatoes, coarsely chopped

2 tablespoons sugar

8-ounce package of whole wheat lasagna noodles (I use Westbrae Natural brand)

1 cup fresh basil leaves (about ¾ ounces), torn, stems removed

1 cup shredded part-skim mozzarella cheese

¼ cup shredded Parmesan cheese

Preheat oven to 400°F. Spray a large (9"×13") rectangular lasagna pan with nonstick cooking spray. Remove ends of eggplants and cut lengthwise into ½-inch slices. Arrange eggplant slices in a colander and sprinkle with salt until slices are lightly covered. Let stand for approximately 15 minutes. In the meantime, add ½ tablespoon olive oil to a large skillet and fry mushrooms and garlic over medium-high heat until mushrooms are well browned and water has evaporated. Remove from pan and set aside. Rinse off salt from eggplant and pat dry. Add ½ tablespoon olive oil to skillet and fry eggplant slices over medium-high heat, in batches (adding in olive oil as needed), until eggplant is soft and browned on both sides. Set browned eggplant aside. In a separate mixing bowl, blend together canned tomatoes, tomato paste, fresh tomatoes, and sugar and set aside. Layer a large lasagna pan with three noodles followed by half of eggplant, half of mushroom mixture, half of basil leaves, a third of the mozzarella cheese, and a third of the tomato sauce. Cover with another layer of noodles and top with the rest of the eggplant, mushrooms, basil, and another third of the mozzarella cheese, and another third of the tomato sauce. Cover with a final layer of noodles and top with remaining tomato sauce and mozzarella cheese. Bake for 40 minutes, uncovered. Sprinkle Parmesan cheese on top before serving.

Nutritional information per serving (⅛ of lasagna, 372 grams):

Calories: 278, Fat: 9 g, Cholesterol: 9 mg, Sodium: 580 mg, Carbohydrate: 40 g, Dietary Fiber: 6 g, Sugars: 9 g, Protein: 13 g

Wednesday's Recipes

Bean Quesadillas

YIELD: 4 SERVINGS

1 teaspoon olive oil

½ cup chopped onion

2 garlic cloves, chopped

1 can (15 ounces) black beans, rinsed and drained

½ red pepper, chopped

3 plum tomatoes, chopped into small pieces

½ pound frozen sweet corn kernels

¼ teaspoon salt

¼ teaspoon pepper

Filling:

In a large skillet, add olive oil, onion, and garlic and sauté over medium-high heat until onion is translucent and lightly browned. Add beans, red pepper, tomatoes, corn, salt, and pepper and heat until mixture has warmed and corn has defrosted (about 5 minutes), stirring occasionally.

One quesadilla:

¼ cup Veggie Shreds soy cheese, cheddar flavor

1 large 100% whole wheat flour tortilla

Taco sauce, optional

Take one large flour tortilla, add ¼ of the bean mixture, and top with ¼ cup shredded soy cheese. Roll tortilla and heat in microwave until cheese melts, about 30 seconds. Top with your favorite taco sauce and enjoy!

Nutritional information per serving (1 quesadilla with ¼ of filling recipe and one tablespoon taco sauce):

Calories: 400, Fat: 8 g, Cholesterol: 0 mg, Sodium: 1042 mg, Carbohydrate: 57 g, Dietary Fiber: 9 g, Sugars: 9 g, Protein: 23 g

Mandarin Orange Almond Salad

Dressing:

¼ cup canola oil

⅛ teaspoon almond extract

2 tablespoons sugar

2 tablespoons balsamic vinegar

1 tablespoon white vinegar

2 tablespoons juice (syrup) from canned mandarin oranges

¼ teaspoon salt

In a bowl, combine all dressing ingredients and whisk until blended. Chill dressing until serving salad.

Salad:

YIELD: 2 SERVINGS

3 tablespoons sliced green onions

1 cup chopped green pepper

4 cups mixed greens (I use Earthbound Farm organically grown mixed baby greens)

½ cup slivered almonds

1 can (11 ounces) mandarin oranges in light syrup

Place greens in salad bowl; add green onions and green pepper. Toss. Decorate with almonds and drained oranges before serving. Add desired amount of salad dressing and toss.

Nutritional information per serving (½ of salad recipe with approximately 2 tablespoons salad dressing):

Calories: 349, Fat: 23 g, Cholesterol: 0 mg, Sodium: 137 mg, Carbohydrate: 31 g, Dietary Fiber: 6 g, Sugars: 9 g, Protein: 10 g

Shrimp and Tofu Stir Fry

YIELD: 4 SERVINGS

2 tablespoons canola oil

1 pound large shrimp, peeled and cleaned (with tails on)

4 garlic cloves, minced

2 tablespoons fresh, peeled ginger, minced

1 package (14 ounces) super-firm cubed tofu, drained

1 can (8 ounces) pineapple tidbits, in juice, drained

12 ounces fresh green beans, trimmed

⅓ cup organic reduced-sodium chicken broth

3 tablespoons teriyaki sauce

3 green onions, thinly sliced

Heat 1 tablespoon canola oil in a large skillet, over medium-high heat. Add shrimp and fry for approximately 5 minutes, stirring frequently and flipping sides, until shrimp has turned opaque. Transfer shrimp to a plate. Add another tablespoon of canola oil to skillet. Add garlic, ginger, and tofu, and sauté until garlic and tofu are light brown in color, about 5 minutes. Add pineapple and sauté until the pineapple takes on a caramelized appearance. Add green beans to the skillet and cook an additional 5 minutes, turning frequently. Return shrimp, then add chicken broth and teriyaki sauce, and stir. Cover and cook until green beans are crisp, about 5 minutes. Remove from heat, stir in green onions, and serve immediately with a side of brown rice (topped with Benecol Light Spread).

Nutritional information per serving (¼ of recipe, 369 grams or approximately 1½ cups):

Calories: 290, Fat: 10 g, Cholesterol: 173 mg, Sodium: 715 mg, Carbohydrate: 18 g, Dietary Fiber: 4 g, Sugars: 11 g, Protein: 30 g

Thursday's Recipes

Walnut Hummus and Vegetable Sandwich Wrap

YIELD: 14 SERVINGS

1 large garlic clove

½ cup chopped walnuts, toasted

Juice from 1 lemon

1 can (15 ounces) garbanzo beans, rinsed and drained

½ cup tahini

½ teaspoon sea salt

½ cup water

Filling:

In a food processor, chop garlic into small pieces. Toast walnuts on a tray lined with aluminum foil in a toaster oven at 300°F until golden brown (shaking pan frequently to prevent scorching), about 5 minutes. Add walnuts, lemon juice, garbanzo beans, tahini, salt, and water to food processor and process until smooth. Serve hummus as a sandwich stuffer or as a dip for crudités.

One sandwich:1 large 100% whole wheat wrap

Chopped spinach, tomatoes, red onions, roasted red peppers, or vegetables of your choice

Take a 100 percent whole wheat wrap and spread it on a cutting board. Spread ¼ cup hummus on the wrap. Add chopped spinach, tomatoes, red onions, roasted red peppers, and any other type of vegetable that you desire. Roll the wrap tightly, cut in half, and serve.

Nutritional information per serving (1 vegetable sandwich wrap with 1 cup assorted raw vegetables and 55 grams hummus or approximately ¼ cup):

Calories: 318, Fat: 11 g, Cholesterol: 0 mg, Sodium: 314 mg, Carbohydrate: 49 g, Dietary Fiber: 6 g, Sugars: 3 g, Protein: 13 g

Smoky Baba Ghanoush

YIELD: 14 SERVINGS

2 large eggplants

3 tablespoons olive oil

½ cup onions, chopped

4 garlic cloves, minced

1 cup tomatoes, chopped

2 garlic cloves, chopped

Juice from 1 lemon

2 tablespoons tahini

2 tablespoons plain nonfat yogurt

½ teaspoon salt

Dash of freshly ground pepper

Pinch of ground cumin

Cut the ends off the eggplants and slice lengthwise, cutting almost all the way through so that eggplant halves fan open. Place each eggplant on enough aluminum foil so that you can close the foil around the eggplant and create a closed cooking pouch. Spread ½ tablespoon olive oil on each eggplant half. Add half the onion and 2 minced garlic cloves to each eggplant. Seal the aluminum foil and place on a grill, cooking over medium-high heat until the flesh of the eggplant is soft, about 40 minutes. Remove from grill and aluminum foil and cool. Scoop out the cooked eggplant flesh and place in a food processor with the onions and garlic. Add remaining ingredients (tomatoes, garlic, lemon juice, tahini, olive oil, yogurt, salt, pepper, and cumin) and process until smooth. Serve with pita chips or warmed whole wheat pita, either at room temperature or chilled.

Nutritional information per serving (1⁄14 of recipe, 102 grams or approximately ¼ cup):

Calories: 67, Fat: 4 g, Cholesterol: 0 mg, Sodium: 88 mg, Carbohydrate: 7 g, Dietary Fiber: 0 g, Sugars: 1 g, Protein: 1 g

Bean Brownies

YIELD: 12 SERVINGS

1 can (15 ounces) black beans, unseasoned

1 box prepared brownie mix

1 cup (4 ounces) unsweetened applesauce

⅓ cup semi-sweet chocolate mini morsels

Preheat oven to 300°F. Spray a 9"×13" rectangular baking pan with nonstick cooking spray. In a food processor, puree the black beans (use entire can, liquid and all). In a large mixing bowl, add brownie mix, applesauce, mini morsels, and bean puree and blend well until smooth. Spread mix into baking pan and bake until brownie springs back when lightly touched, about 35 minutes. Cool and serve with fat-free whipped topping, if desired.

Nutritional information per serving (1 brownie, 1⁄12 of recipe, 92 grams):

Calories: 217, Fat: 2 g, Cholesterol: 0 mg, Sodium: 350 mg, Carbohydrate: 46 g, Dietary Fiber: 2 g, Sugars: 29 g, Protein: 3 g

Friday's Recipes

Egg White Omelet with Cheese

YIELD: 1 SERVING

Canola oil nonstick cooking spray

3 egg whites

2 slices mozzarella-flavored soy cheese

Coat a skillet with nonstick cooking spray and bring to medium-high heat. In a bowl, whisk egg whites until slight foam forms. Pour egg whites into preheated skillet. Cook egg whites until firm and place cheese slices in center of omelet. Fold egg whites over with a spatula and flip. Cook until omelet is the desired consistency. Serve immediately with 2 soy sausages, 100 percent whole wheat toast, and Benecol Light Spread, if desired.

Nutritional information per serving (one omelet):

Calories: 134, Fat: 4 g, Cholesterol: 0 mg, Sodium: 686 mg, Carbohydrate: 3 g, Dietary Fiber: 0 g, Sugars: 1 g, Protein: 19 g

Vanilla Soy Smoothie with Flaxseeds

YIELD: 1 SERVING

8 ounces light vanilla soy milk

2 tablespoons ground flaxseeds

½ cup frozen peaches (no added sugar)

2 tablespoons sugar

Add all ingredients into a blender and process until smooth.

Nutritional information per serving (approximately 13 fluid ounces):

Calories: 285, Fat: 8 g, Cholesterol: 0 mg, Sodium: 100 mg, Carbohydrate: 50 g, Dietary Fiber: 5 g, Sugars: 28 g, Protein: 7 g

Spinach Salad

YIELD: 4 SERVINGS

Dressing:

¼ cup red wine vinegar

¼ teaspoon balsamic vinegar

Juice from 1 lemon

Dash pepper

1 tablespoon Dijon mustard

¼ cup 100% pure maple syrup

¼ cup canola oil

In a food processor, process all ingredients except oil until blended. Slowly pour oil into food processor, pulsing until well blended. Chill until salad is served.

Salad:

½ cup chopped walnuts

6 cups organic baby spinach leaves

1 green apple, cored and thinly sliced

1 ripe pear, cored and thinly sliced

4 teaspoons gorgonzola cheese, crumbled

Preheat a toaster oven to 350°F. Spread walnuts on an aluminum foil–covered baking pan. Toast walnuts for approximately 3 minutes, shaking pan occasionally to prevent scorching. Place spinach, apple and pear slices, and walnuts in a salad bowl and toss. Serve salad in salad bowls and sprinkle each with 1 teaspoon gorgonzola cheese and 1 tablespoon dressing and serve.

Nutritional information per serving (¼ of salad plus 1 tablespoon of salad dressing):

Calories: 208, Fat: 15 g, Cholesterol: 2 mg, Sodium: 155 mg, Carbohydrate: 21 g, Dietary Fiber: 5 g, Sugars: 11 g, Protein: 4 g

Chicken with 40 Cloves of Garlic

YIELD: 8 SERVINGS

2½–3 pounds skinless chicken parts (preferably free-range chicken raised without antibiotics or hormones)

3 tablespoons extra virgin olive oil

1 teaspoon salt

1 teaspoon pepper

40 garlic cloves

12-ounce package of sliced white mushrooms

1 pound red potatoes, washed, scrubbed, and halved

2 whole medium onions

2 cups burgundy cooking wine

2 cups organic reduced-sodium chicken broth

1 sprig fresh rosemary

3 sprigs fresh thyme

Preheat oven to 350°F. Rinse chicken and pat dry. In a large skillet, heat 2 tablespoons olive oil over medium-high heat. Add chicken parts and season with salt and pepper on both sides. Sauté chicken on both sides until just brown. Remove chicken from skillet and place in a large baking dish suitable for cooking in the oven. In the same skillet, add the 40 cloves of garlic and cook in the oil and juice from the chicken until brown on both sides. Add garlic to baking dish. Add mushrooms to skillet and cook over medium-high heat until much of the water has evaporated and the mushrooms are brown. Remove mushrooms and add to the baking dish. Add one tablespoon olive oil into skillet, add potatoes, and cook over medium-high heat until both sides are brown. Add potatoes to baking dish. Add onions, burgundy wine, chicken broth, rosemary, and thyme to baking dish. Cover and place in oven. Cook for 60 minutes, basting once during cooking.

Nutritional information per serving (⅛ of recipe, 448 grams or approximately 2 cups):

Calories: 376, Fat: 8 g, Cholesterol: 100 mg, Sodium: 915 mg, Carbohydrate: 29 g, Dietary Fiber: 2 g, Sugars: 5 g, Protein: 43 g

Barley Risotto with Shiitake Mushrooms

YIELD: 6 SERVINGS

1 container (32 fluid ounces) free-range organic chicken broth

1 bay leaf

½ teaspoon thyme

1 tablespoon extra virgin olive oil

1 cup chopped onion

2 garlic cloves, minced

1 cup whole-grain barley

1 package (10 ounces) frozen shiitake mushrooms, defrosted (I use Woodstock Farms organic shiitake mushrooms, available in the frozen foods section of your local health food store)

½ teaspoon salt

¼ teaspoon freshly ground black pepper

⅓ cup freshly shredded Parmesan cheese

In a small saucepan, heat chicken broth, bay leaf, and thyme and bring to a simmer. Let simmer while preparing barley. In a large saucepan, heat olive oil over medium-high heat. Add onions and garlic and sauté until onion is translucent, approximately 3 minutes. Add barley and package of mushrooms and cook an additional 5 minutes, stirring frequently. Add chicken broth and simmer, covered, until most of the broth has evaporated and the barley is tender, about 45 minutes. Season with salt and pepper, add the Parmesan cheese, stir, and serve immediately.

Nutritional information per serving (⅙ of recipe, 277 grams or approximately 1¼ cups):

Calories: 128, Fat: 5 g, Cholesterol: 6 mg, Sodium: 577 mg, Carbohydrate: 17 g, Dietary Fiber: 4 g, Sugars: 2 g, Protein: 6 g

Okra Succotash

YIELD: 6 SERVINGS

3 large ripe tomatoes

3 cups frozen, sliced okra (defrosted)

1 teaspoon salt

¼ teaspoon freshly ground black pepper

2 cups frozen baby lima beans (defrosted)

2 cups frozen sweet corn kernels (defrosted)

4 tablespoons Benecol Light Spread

Spray a large saucepan with nonstick cooking spray. Cut tomatoes up into small pieces. Add tomatoes, okra, salt, and pepper to saucepan, cover, and simmer over low heat for 10 minutes, stirring occasionally. Add lima beans and simmer, covered, for an additional 15 minutes. Add corn kernels, stir, and simmer, covered, for 5 more minutes. Add Benecol and stir. Serve immediately.

Nutritional information per serving (⅙ of recipe, 219 grams or approximately 1 cup):

Calories: 181, Fat: 5 g, Cholesterol: 0 mg, Sodium: 572 mg, Carbohydrate: 29 g, Dietary Fiber: 6 g, Sugars: 4 g, Protein: 8 g

Saturday's Recipes

Falafel Pita Pockets with Yogurt and Dill Sauce

YIELD: 4 SERVINGS

Falafel:

1 box (10 ounces) falafel mix

1¼ cups water

4 tablespoons canola oil

In a large mixing bowl, combine 1 packet of falafel mix with water. Blend well and let stand 10 minutes. In the meantime, heat 2 tablespoons canola oil in a large skillet (swirl to coat pan), until oil is hot enough that a droplet of water sizzles. Shape falafel mixture into small, round, approximately 1-inch balls. Drop in oil (be careful not to splatter the hot oil!) and fry in batches, adding more oil as necessary, until golden brown on both sides, about 4 minutes. Remove and place on paper towels to soak up excess oil.

Tahini sauce:

2 garlic cloves, minced

⅓ cup tahini

1 tablespoon extra virgin olive oil

Juice from 1 lemon

¼ cup water

¼ teaspoon salt

In a food processor, mince garlic cloves. Add tahini, olive oil, lemon juice, water, and salt and puree until mixture is well blended. Mixture should be thin and pourable.

Yogurt sauce:

1 garlic clove

1 cup nonfat plain yogurt

2 teaspoons extra virgin olive oil

Juice from ½ lemon

1 tablespoon chopped fresh dill

In a food processor, mince garlic clove. Add yogurt and olive oil and pulse until blended. Add lemon juice and pulse again until mixture is blended. Pour mixture into serving dish, add dill, and stir to blend.

Pita pockets:

2 large whole wheat pita breads

½ cup peeled and chopped cucumber

½ cup chopped tomato

1 cup shredded lettuce (I use spinach, for the most nutrition)

Cut whole wheat pita bread in half to make 2 pockets. Pour 1 or 2 tablespoons of tahini sauce inside each pita half. Fill each pocket with falafel, cucumber, tomato, and spinach. Top with 2 tablespoons yogurt sauce and serve.

Nutritional information per serving (1 pita pocket with ¼ falafel mixture, ¼ vegetables, 2 tablespoons tahini, and 2 tablespoons yogurt sauce):

Calories: 428, Fat: 21 g, Cholesterol: 1 mg, Sodium: 607 mg, Carbohydrate: 50 g, Dietary Fiber: 8 g, Sugars: 7 g, Protein: 14 g

Butternut Squash French Fries

YIELD: 2 SERVINGS

2 large butternut squash

Canola oil nonstick cooking spray

1 teaspoon salt

Preheat oven to 425°F. Peel squash with a vegetable peeler. With a sharp knife, cut off the ends and slice in half. Remove the seeds and continue to slice squash up into small French fry shapes. Spray a large nonstick cookie sheet with canola cooking spray. Arrange fries on sheet in a single layer. Spray fries with canola spray and then sprinkle evenly with salt. Bake for 40 minutes, turning once. Fries should be crispy and brown at the edges. Serve right out of the oven.

Nutritional information per serving (½ of recipe, 243 grams or approximately 1 cup):

Calories: 109, Fat: 0 g, Cholesterol: 0 mg, Sodium: 1172 mg, Carbohydrate: 28 g, Dietary Fiber: 5 g, Sugars: 5 g, Protein: 2 g

Garlicky Bean Dip

YIELD: 10 SERVINGS

1 can (15.5 ounces) cannellini beans, rinsed and drained

⅓ cup extra virgin olive oil

1 garlic clove, minced

½ teaspoon salt

Juice from ½ lemon

Freshly ground black pepper

In a food processor, add beans, olive oil, and minced garlic. Process until smooth. Season with salt, lemon juice and pepper, blend, and transfer mixture to a serving dish. Serve as a dip for fresh vegetables or as a spread on a baked tortilla or whole wheat pita chips.

Nutritional information per serving (1/10 of recipe, 54 grams or approximately ¼ cup):

Calories: 97, Fat: 8 g, Cholesterol: 0 mg, Sodium: 275 mg, Carbohydrate: 7 g, Dietary Fiber: 2 g, Sugars: 0 g, Protein: 3 g

Sunday's Recipes

Oat-Apple-Flax Pancakes

YIELD: 6 SERVINGS

1 cup old-fashioned oats

½ cup flour

⅓ cup ground flaxseeds

4 tablespoons sugar

1 tablespoon baking powder

½ teaspoon salt

¼ teaspoon cinnamon

¼ teaspoon nutmeg

3 egg whites, stiffly beaten

1¼ cup light soy milk

1 tablespoon canola oil

1 cup shredded apple

In a food processor, process oats into a fine flour-like consistency. In a large bowl, combine oat flour, flour, flaxseeds, sugar, baking powder, salt, cinnamon, and nutmeg. In a separate bowl, whisk egg whites until foamy and set aside. In another bowl, mix together soy milk and oil and add to flour mixture. In the food processor, chop the apple into small pieces and add to flour mixture. Fold in egg mixture and stir all ingredients until just combined. On a hot griddle coated with canola oil, pour approximately ¼ cup of batter for each pancake and cook until bubbles appear. Flip pancake and cook until just brown. Serve warm and garnish with Benecol Light Spread, pure maple syrup, and chopped almonds, if desired.

Nutritional information per serving (⅙ of recipe, 152 grams pancake batter or approximately ¾ cup batter making 3 pancakes):

Calories: 320, Fat: 10 g, Cholesterol: 0 mg, Sodium: 667 mg, Carbohydrate: 51 g, Dietary Fiber: 6 g, Sugars: 17 g, Protein: 10 g

Tuna Salad

YIELD: 4 SERVINGS

Dressing:

¼ cup extra virgin olive oil

¼ cup red wine vinegar

Juice from 1 lemon

4 garlic cloves, chopped into small pieces

In a bowl, combine all dressing ingredients and whisk until blended. Place in large salad bowl.

Salad:

1 small red onion, halved and thinly sliced

1 red pepper, thinly sliced

1 can (12.5 ounces) white tuna in water, drained and flaked

½ cup sliced black olives

1 cup chickpeas, rinsed and drained

¼ cup fresh chopped parsley

¼ teaspoon salt

¼ teaspoon pepper

2 bags (4 ounces each) organic mixed baby greens

Add onion, pepper, tuna, olives, chickpeas, parsley, and salt and pepper to the salad bowl containing the dressing. Toss until mixed thoroughly. Place greens on a serving plate, dish out tuna salad onto greens, and serve.

Nutritional information per serving (¼ of recipe, 346 grams or approximately 1½ cups salad):

Calories: 348, Fat: 18 g, Cholesterol: 26 mg, Sodium: 682 mg, Carbohydrate: 21 g, Dietary Fiber: 5 g, Sugars: 2 g, Protein: 27 g

Arugula Salad with Garlic Tomato Vinaigrette

YIELD: 4 SERVINGS

Dressing:

Two fresh basil leaves, shredded

2 tablespoons chopped garlic

4 tablespoons balsamic vinegar

4 tablespoons extra virgin olive oil

1 teaspoon Worcestershire sauce

Juice from 1 lemon

¼ teaspoon salt

¼ teaspoon pepper

3 plum tomatoes, chopped

In a bowl, combine all dressing ingredients (except tomatoes) and whisk until blended. Add tomatoes and blend with vinaigrette. Chill dressing until salad is served.

Salad:

3 cups arugula

1 small head of radicchio, chopped

1 Belgian endive, end cut off and leaves separated

Place greens in salad bowl and toss. Add salad dressing and serve.

Nutritional information per serving (¼ of the salad greens with approximately ¼ cup dressing):

Calories: 145, Fat: 10 g, Cholesterol: 0 mg, Sodium: 149 mg, Carbohydrate: 11 g, Dietary Fiber: 4 g, Sugars: 4 g, Protein: 2 g

Pasta with Meatballs

YIELD: 10 SERVINGS

Homemade tomato sauce:

2 tablespoons extra virgin olive oil

8 ounces white mushrooms, sliced

1 medium onion, chopped

1 large carrot, peeled and thinly sliced

2 large garlic cloves, chopped

1 leek, the white section and 1 inch of the green, cleaned and thinly sliced

2 large basil leaves, shredded

1 can (35 ounces) Italian peeled tomatoes

1 container (26.46 ounces) "Pomi" chopped tomatoes

2 tablespoons sugar

½ teaspoon salt

¼ teaspoon black pepper

In a large saucepan, heat 1 tablespoon olive oil over medium-high heat. Add mushrooms and cook until browned and much of the liquid has evaporated. Remove mushrooms and set aside. Add remaining olive oil and heat over medium-high heat. Sauté onion, carrot, garlic, leek, and basil leaves until carrots are soft, about 6 minutes. Stir in tomatoes. In a food processor, add tomato/vegetable mixture and puree in batches. Add sugar, salt, and pepper and place pureed tomato sauce back in saucepan. Heat over medium-high heat until just boiling, reduce to a simmer, and cook uncovered for approximately 30 minutes, stirring occasionally.

Pasta dish:

1 box (16 ounces) 100% whole wheat rotini pasta

1 cup shredded part-skim mozzarella cheese

1 cup mozzarella flavor shredded soy cheese

10 meatless meatballs

Freshly shredded Parmesan cheese

Cook pasta according to package directions. Preheat oven to 350°F. In a large mixing bowl, add pasta, tomato sauce, mozzarella cheese, soy cheese, and meatballs. Mix and pour into a very large baking dish (I use a large lasagna pan). Bake uncovered in oven until cheese melts, about 20 minutes. Serve warm, sprinkled with fresh Parmesan cheese.

Nutritional information per serving (1⁄10 of recipe, 338 grams or approximately 1½ cups pasta with 1 tablespoon Parmesan cheese):

Calories: 491, Fat: 16 g, Cholesterol: 9 mg, Sodium: 1113 mg, Carbohydrate: 56 g, Dietary Fiber: 9 g, Sugars: 10 g, Protein: 34 g

Roasted Baby Eggplant with Tomatoes

YIELD: 8 SERVINGS

4 baby eggplants

8 plum tomatoes, sliced lengthwise

4 garlic cloves, thinly sliced

¼ cup extra virgin olive oil

½ cup balsamic vinegar

½ teaspoon salt

½ teaspoon pepper

Preheat oven to 400°F. Trim and discard stalks from the eggplants. Slice eggplant into quarters, lengthwise. Spray a roasting dish with nonstick spray. Put eggplant, tomatoes, and garlic into roasting dish. Drizzle oil and vinegar over vegetables, and salt and pepper to taste. Roast in oven for 1 hour (turn once to prevent charring). Serve hot.

Nutritional information per serving (⅛ of recipe, 223 grams or approximately 1 cup):

Calories: 121, Fat: 8 g, Cholesterol: 0 mg, Sodium: 158 mg, Carbohydrate: 14 g, Dietary Fiber: 1 g, Sugars: 4 g, Protein: 2 g

Chocolate Almond Decadence

YIELD: 12 SERVINGS

Cake:

6 squares Baker's unsweetened baking chocolate

¾ cup Benecol Light Spread

2 cups sugar

½ cup flour

½ cup almond flour (almonds ground into a fine powder)

1 cup (4 ounces) unsweetened applesauce

3 egg whites

1 teaspoon vanilla extract

½ cup Nestlé Toll House semi-sweet chocolate mini morsels

Preheat oven to 350°F. Spray a 9"×13" baking pan with nonstick cooking spray and set aside. Combine the first two ingredients in a large microwavable bowl and microwave on high for 2 minutes. Remove and stir until chocolate is completely melted. In another large mixing bowl, combine sugar, flour, and almond flour (process raw, natural almonds in a food processor until almonds are a fine powder). Add the remaining ingredients and mix well until completely blended. Pour batter into baking pan and bake until center is firm to the touch, about 35 minutes. Let stand until set and serve warm, topped with raspberry coulis and fat-free whipped topping, if desired.

Raspberry coulis:

2½ cups fresh raspberries

⅓ cup sugar

1 teaspoon fresh lemon juice

In a saucepan, add raspberries, sugar, and lemon juice and cook over low heat, stirring gently until sugar is dissolved. When mixture is just beginning to simmer, remove from heat and pour into a food processor. Process until smooth. Drizzle coulis over chocolate almond cake, add a dollop of fat-free Cool Whip, and enjoy!

Nutritional information per serving (1 piece of cake [1⁄12 of recipe, 98 grams] with 2 tablespoons raspberry coulis):

Calories: 378, Fat: 19 g, Cholesterol: 0 mg, Sodium: 125 mg, Carbohydrate: 57 g, Dietary Fiber: 5 g, Sugars: 45 g, Protein: 5 g

Bonus Recipes

Roasted Vegetable Medley

YIELD: 4 SERVINGS

2 tablespoons extra virgin olive oil

½ tablespoon soy sauce

Freshly ground black pepper

1 bag (12 ounces) "Eat Smart" vegetable medley (broccoli, cauliflower, carrots) (available in produce section of some supermarkets)

6 garlic cloves, sliced

Preheat oven to 450°F. Spray a baking sheet with nonstick spray. In a large mixing bowl, combine olive oil, soy sauce, and black pepper. Whisk together until blended. Add the vegetable medley and garlic and stir to coat. Spread veggies in a single layer on baking sheet. Roast vegetables until browned, about 10 minutes. Serve warm.

Nutritional information per serving (¼ of recipe, 99 grams or approximately ½ cup):

Calories: 124, Fat: 7 g, Cholesterol: 0 mg, Sodium: 202 mg, Carbohydrate: 13 g, Dietary Fiber: 3 g, Sugars: 3 g, Protein: 3 g

Bean Salad

YIELD: 6 SERVINGS

SALAD:

1 can (15 ounces) red kidney beans, rinsed and drained

1 can (15 ounces) chickpeas, rinsed and drained

2 cups chopped fresh tomatoes

1 large cucumber, peeled and chopped

1 cup frozen corn kernels

1 cup diced red onion

DRESSING:

4 tablespoons extra virgin olive oil

2 teaspoons Dijon mustard

2 tablespoons balsamic vinegar

Juice from 1 lemon

2 garlic cloves, minced

¼ teaspoon freshly ground black pepper

In a large mixing bowl, combine beans, chickpeas, tomatoes, cucumber, corn, and onion and set aside. In a separate mixing bowl, combine olive oil, mustard, vinegar, lemon juice, garlic, and pepper and whisk together until blended. Pour dressing into bean mixture and toss to combine. Cover and refrigerate until chilled.

Nutritional information per serving (⅙ of recipe, 328 grams or approximately 1½ cups):

Calories: 288, Fat: 11 g, Cholesterol: 0 mg, Sodium: 258 mg, Carbohydrate: 39 g, Dietary Fiber: 11 g, Sugars: 7 g, Protein: 11 g

Ratatouille

YIELD: 12 SERVINGS

5 tablespoons extra virgin olive oil

2 pounds or 2 cans (28 ounces each) whole tomatoes, peeled, drained, and chopped

½ teaspoon salt

½ teaspoon pepper

1 bay leaf

1 teaspoon fresh rosemary, chopped

1 teaspoon fresh thyme, chopped

4 large garlic cloves, minced

1 large onion, halved and sliced

1 red pepper, cut into half-inch strips

1 green pepper, cut into half-inch strips

4 small zucchini, cut into half-inch slices

1 eggplant, diced into one-inch cubes

½ teaspoon salt

½ teaspoon pepper

1 tablespoon sugar

2 tablespoons fresh basil, chopped

In a large skillet, heat 1 tablespoon oil. Add tomatoes, salt, pepper, and bay leaf and bring to a boil over medium-high heat. Reduce heat to a simmer and cook for 15 minutes. Remove bay leaf, add rosemary and thyme, stir, and continue to simmer. In the meantime, in another large skillet, heat 2 tablespoons oil. Add garlic and onions and sauté over low heat for 5 minutes. Add red and green peppers and continue to cook an additional 7 minutes over medium heat. Add zucchini and continue to sauté for 5 additional minutes. In the meantime, in a large Dutch oven (or a stockpot with a lid), heat 2 tablespoons oil and add eggplant cubes and additional salt and pepper. Cook over medium heat for 3 minutes. Add zucchini and pepper mixture to eggplant and cook over medium heat for 7 minutes. Add tomato mixture and sugar, stir, and bring to a boil over medium-high heat. Reduce heat to a simmer, cover, and cook for an additional 5 minutes. Uncover and cook 5 more minutes until tender. Stir in basil and serve.

Nutritional information per serving (1⁄12 of recipe, 240 grams or approximately 1 cup):

Calories: 109, Fat: 6 g, Cholesterol: 0 mg, Sodium: 439 mg, Carbohydrate: 12 g, Dietary Fiber: 2 g, Sugars: 6 g, Protein: 2 g

Red Snapper with Tomatoes and Capers

YIELD: 4 SERVINGS

1 tablespoon extra virgin olive oil

1 onion, cut in half and sliced

4 garlic cloves, thinly sliced

2 cans (14.5 ounces each) diced tomatoes

2 tablespoons drained capers

8 kalamata olives, pitted and sliced

Juice from ½ lemon

1 teaspoon dried basil

1 teaspoon dried oregano

Freshly ground black pepper (I use ¼ teaspoon)

4 red snapper fillets, about 6 ounces each

Preheat oven to 450°F. In a large skillet, add olive oil and heat over medium-high heat. Add onion and garlic and cook until onion is translucent and slightly brown. Add tomatoes, capers, olives, lemon juice, and spices and stir. Bring to a boil, then reduce heat and simmer 5 minutes. In the meantime, spray a large baking dish with nonstick cooking spray. Add fish to baking dish. Top fish with tomato mixture and bake uncovered until fish flakes easily with a fork, about 10 minutes.

Nutritional information per serving (¼ of recipe, 438 grams or 1 snapper fillet with approximately 1 cup sauce):

Calories: 281, Fat: 8 g, Cholesterol: 63 mg, Sodium: 921 mg, Carbohydrate: 15 g, Dietary Fiber: 1 g, Sugars: 8 g, Protein: 38 g

Grilled Salmon with Lentil and Root Vegetable Ragout

YIELD: 4 SERVINGS

1 cup French lentils, washed and picked over

1 small onion, peeled and with a clove inserted

1 small carrot, peeled and cut in half

5 sprigs fresh parsley

2 sprigs fresh thyme

1 large bay leaf

2 tablespoons extra virgin olive oil

1 large carrot, peeled, quartered, and diced into ¼-inch pieces

2 turnips, peeled and diced into ½-inch pieces

¼ teaspoon salt

⅛ teaspoon pepper

2 shallots, finely minced

4 medium-sized garlic cloves, minced

4 tablespoons extra virgin olive oil

4 center-cut wild salmon fillets, about 6 ounces each

1 teaspoon salt

½ teaspoon black pepper

Fresh lemon wedges and parsley, for garnish

Lentils:

In a large mixing bowl, rinse lentils with water. In a large saucepan, add drained lentils, onion, carrot, parsley, thyme, and bay leaf. Cover with water (approximately 2 inches above lentils) and bring to a boil. Reduce heat and simmer, covered, stirring occasionally, until lentils are tender, about 30 minutes. Reserve ¾ cup cooking liquid and drain the rest. Discard vegetables and herbs and set cooked lentils aside.

Vegetables:

Heat the olive oil in a large skillet over medium-high heat. Add carrots and turnips, season with salt and pepper, and cook, stirring occasionally, for approximately 10 minutes. Transfer to a plate and add shallot and garlic to skillet and cook until lightly browned, about 2 minutes. Add back lentils, vegetables, and lentil broth. Cover and simmer until broth has been absorbed, about 15 minutes. Keep warm until salmon has been cooked.

Salmon:

Preheat grill to high heat. Rinse salmon and pat dry. Pour a small amount of olive oil on top side of each fillet and coat lightly. Sprinkle both sides with salt and pepper to taste. Grill salmon, skin side up, until fish is no longer pink on the inside and flakes easily with a fork, about 10 minutes. Flip and cook an additional few minutes until skin is crispy. Serve salmon immediately, placed on a bed of lentil and vegetable ragout. Garnish with fresh lemon and parsley.

Nutritional information per serving (1 salmon fillet with approximately 1 cup lentil and vegetable ragout):

Calories: 628, Fat: 32 g, Cholesterol: 94 mg, Sodium: 889 mg, Carbohydrate: 38 g, Dietary Fiber: 9 g, Sugars: 7 g, Protein: 46 g

Mixed Vegetable Curry

YIELD: 8 SERVINGS

2 teaspoons canola oil

2 teaspoons coriander

½ teaspoon chili powder

¼ teaspoon turmeric

1-inch piece of fresh ginger, peeled and grated

1 large onion, chopped

2 garlic cloves, crushed

1 small cauliflower, cut into florets

2 potatoes, cut into small cubes

2 carrots, sliced

1 green pepper, cored, seeded, and cut into small chunks

1 fresh green chili, cored, seeded, and finely chopped

1 can (14.5 ounces) whole, peeled tomatoes (chopped into quarters)

⅔ cup light coconut milk (I use A Taste of Thai brand Lite Coconut Milk)

1 teaspoon salt

½ teaspoon black pepper

Juice from ½ lemon

Heat oil over medium heat in a large stockpot. Add coriander, chili powder, and turmeric and cook for 1 minute. Add ginger, onion, and garlic to the pot and cook until the onion is softened but not browned, about 5 minutes. Add cauliflower, potatoes, and carrots and stir to coat with the spices. Cook an additional 5 minutes. Add the green pepper, chili, can of tomatoes (do not drain), coconut milk, salt, and pepper and stir well. Bring to a boil, cover, and simmer for 30 minutes, stirring occasionally. Stir in lemon juice and serve immediately.

Nutritional information per serving (serving size: ⅛ of recipe, 198 grams or approximately 1 cup):

Calories: 103, Fat: 3 g, Cholesterol: 0 mg, Sodium: 414 mg, Carbohydrate: 18 g, Dietary Fiber: 3 g, Sugars: 5 g, Protein: 3 g

Coconut Lentils

YIELD: 12 SERVINGS

1 tablespoon extra virgin olive oil

1 cup chopped onions

2 cups lentils, washed and picked over

1 can (400 ml) light coconut milk (I use A Taste of Thai brand Lite Coconut Milk)

2 cups water

1 bay leaf

1 teaspoon salt

¼ teaspoon black pepper

Heat oil over medium heat in a large skillet. Add chopped onions and sauté until onions are lightly browned, about 5 minutes. Add lentils, coconut milk, water, and bay leaf. Stir and bring to a boil. Cover, reduce heat, and simmer for 60 minutes, stirring occasionally. Remove and discard bay leaf, add salt and pepper, and stir. Serve warm.

Nutritional information per serving (serving size: 1⁄12 of recipe, 118 grams or approximately ½ cup):

Calories: 135, Fat: 3 g, Cholesterol: 0 mg, Sodium: 213 mg, Carbohydrate: 21 g, Dietary Fiber: 5 g, Sugars: 2 g, Protein: 8 g

Garlic and White Bean Salad

YIELD: 6 SERVINGS

DRESSING:

¼ cup extra virgin olive oil

1 sprig fresh rosemary

4 large garlic cloves, smashed

3 anchovy fillets, rinsed and patted dry, then chopped into small pieces

¼ cup shredded fresh Parmesan cheese

1 teaspoon grated lemon zest

¼ teaspoon kosher salt

¼ teaspoon black pepper

Juice from 1 lemon

SALAD:

2 cans (15.5 ounces each) cannellini beans, rinsed and drained

2 large, ripe tomatoes, quartered

2 tablespoons freshly chopped parsley

Fresh lemon wedges for garnish

In a small skillet, combine olive oil, rosemary, and garlic. Over moderate heat, cook until rosemary starts to sizzle. Remove from heat and let stand for 30 minutes (so the oil takes on the flavor of garlic and rosemary). Discard rosemary and set infused oil aside. In a food processor, add garlic (removed from the reserved oil), anchovy fillets, Parmesan cheese, lemon zest, salt, pepper, and lemon juice. Process until mixture is well blended. In a large salad bowl, add beans and parsley. Add the dressing and mix beans gently. Add reserved olive oil and tomatoes. Gently stir, cover, and refrigerate for an hour to let beans absorb the flavors. Bring to room temperature and garnish with a few squeezes of fresh lemon juice before serving.

Nutritional information per serving (serving size: ⅙ of recipe, 224 grams or approximately 1 cup):

Calories: 238, Fat: 12 g, Cholesterol: 4 mg, Sodium: 477 mg, Carbohydrate: 24 g, Dietary Fiber: 6 g, Sugars: 2 g, Protein: 9 g

Linguini with Garlicky Clam Sauce

YIELD: 6 SERVINGS

CLAM SAUCE:

½ cup extra virgin olive oil

3 medium onions, chopped

8 large garlic cloves, sliced

1 teaspoon red pepper flakes

¼ teaspoon salt

¼ teaspoon black pepper

2 tablespoons chopped fresh parsley

3 dozen littleneck clams, washed and scrubbed

1 cup white wine

PASTA:

1 box (16 ounces) 100% whole wheat pasta (I use Gia Russa brand imported Italian pasta)

Freshly shredded Parmesan cheese

Cook pasta according to package directions. Heat olive oil in a large skillet, over medium-high heat. Add onions and cook over high heat for 2 minutes.

Reduce heat, add garlic, red pepper flakes, salt, and pepper and simmer, covered, for 45 minutes, stirring frequently. Add parsley, stir, and cook uncovered for 5 more minutes, then set aside.

In a large stockpot, add clams and white wine. Bring to a boil over high heat. Reduce heat to medium, cover, and steam until clams are fully open, about 15 minutes. Remove clams from broth and twist off and discard the top shell, leaving the clam nestled in the bottom shell. Place clams and cooked pasta in a large serving platter. Strain clam broth through a fine sieve to remove any particles. Add clam broth to onion mixture and bring to a boil. Reduce the broth and onion mixture by ¼, stirring frequently. Pour broth over pasta and stir. Serve warm, each serving sprinkled with 1 tablespoon Parmesan cheese.

Nutritional information per serving (serving size: ⅙ of recipe, 308 grams or approximately 1½ cups):

Calories: 588, Fat: 23 g, Cholesterol: 33 mg, Sodium: 396 mg, Carbohydrate: 72 g, Dietary Fiber: 8 g, Sugars: 5 g, Protein: 26 g

Appendix 5

What's Your Risk of Heart Disease?

The NCEP has a simple three-step tool for estimating your risk of developing heart disease.

1. Count Your Major Risk Factors

The top four major risk factors for heart disease according to the American Heart Association are cigarette smoking, high blood pressure, diabetes, and high cholesterol. You should know that they combine exponentially, meaning that two risk factors would increase your risk of contracting cardiovascular disease by significantly more than the amounts of each factor added together.

Risk factors for heart disease were first studied in Framingham, Massachusetts, just outside of Boston. Several generations of families there have shared their personal lifestyle and health information with scientists for over fifty years in what has come to be known as the Framingham Heart Study.[1] This ongoing study identified the risk factors that people who succumbed to cardiovascular disease were likely to share.

Major Risk Factors

Cigarette smoking

High blood pressure (≥140/90 mm Hg or on blood pressure medication)

HDL cholesterol (<40 mg/dL); if HDL is ≥ 60 mg/dL, subtract one risk factor point from your total count)

Family history of early heart disease (in a father or brother < 55 years old; in a mother or sister < 65 years old)

Age (men ≥ 45; women ≥ 55)

My total major risk factor count is ______________.

Source: Adapted from Expert Panel on Detection, Evaluation, and Treatment of High Blood Cholesterol in Adults, "Executive Summary of the Third Report of the National Cholesterol Education Program (NCEP) Expert Panel on Detection, Evaluation, and Treatment of High Blood Cholesterol in Adults (Adult Treatment Panel III)," *JAMA* 285, no. 19 (2001): 2486–2497, https://pubmed.ncbi.nlm.nih.gov/11368702/.

How probable is it that you will suffer a heart attack if you have even one of these four major risk factors? According to a study analyzing data from thousands of individuals who were followed over a period of several decades, 80 to 90 percent of those diagnosed with heart disease and over 95 percent of those who died from the disease had at least one of the four major risk factors.[2] Some risk factors are uncontrollable, such as age, gender, and family history, but there are also some you can control—for example, smoking, a sedentary lifestyle, obesity, and high blood cholesterol. *What is important to understand is that the higher your LDL level and the more risk factors (other than LDL) that you have, the greater your risk of contracting heart or vessel disease.*

2. If You Have More Than Two Major Risk Factors, Take the Framingham 10-Year Risk Assessment

If your major risk factor count totals 2 or more, the NCEP recommends that you proceed to calculate your 10-year risk assessment utilizing the Framingham method of scoring. This is a simple tool for calculating your risk of having a heart attack or stroke over the next 10 years, based on the Framingham Heart Study.

Framingham 10-Year Risk Assessment

The 10-year risk assessment tool is designed for adults who have not been diagnosed with heart disease or diabetes.

10-Year Risk Calculator for Men

1. What is your age?

Age	Points
20–34	–9
35–39	–4
40–44	0
45–49	3
50–54	6
55–59	8

60–64	10
65–69	11
70–74	12
75–79	13

2. What is your HDL cholesterol (mg/dL)?

HDL	Points
≥60	–1
50–59	0
40–49	1
<40	2

3. What is your total cholesterol (mg/dL)?

	Points				
Total Cholesterol:	Age 20–39	Age 40–49	Age 50–59	Age 60–69	Age 70–79
<160	0	0	0	0	0
160–199	4	3	2	1	0
200–239	7	5	3	1	0
240–279	9	6	4	2	1
≥280	11	8	5	3	1

4. Do you smoke?

	Points				
	Age 20–39	Age 40–49	Age 50–59	Age 60–69	Age 70–79
Nonsmoker	0	0	0	0	0
Smoker	8	5	3	1	1

5. What is your blood pressure (mm Hg)?

	Points	
Systolic (top number) BP:	Untreated	Treated with medication
<120	0	0
120–129	0	1
130–139	1	2
140–159	1	2
≥160	2	3

6. What is your 10-year risk?

Points total:	<0–4	5–6	7	8	9	10	11	12	13	14	15	16	≥17
Ten-year risk percentage:	≤1	2	3	4	5	6	8	11	14	17	22	27	≥30

MY 10-YEAR RISK IS ______________ %

10-Year Risk Calculator for Women

1. What is your age?

Age	Points
20–34	–7
35–39	–3
40–44	0
45–49	3
50–54	6
55–59	8

60–64	10
65–69	12
70–74	14
75–79	16

2. What is your HDL cholesterol (mg/dL)?

HDL	Points
≥60	–1
50–59	0
40–49	1
<40	2

3. What is your total cholesterol (mg/dL)?

	Points				
Total Cholesterol:	Age 20–39	Age 40–49	Age 50–59	Age 60–69	Age 70–79
<160	0	0	0	0	0
160–199	4	3	2	1	1
200–239	8	6	4	2	1
240–279	11	8	5	3	2
≥280	13	10	7	4	2

4. Do you smoke?

	Points				
	Age 20–39	Age 40–49	Age 50–59	Age 60–69	Age 70–79
Nonsmoker	0	0	0	0	0
Smoker	9	7	4	2	1

5. What is your blood pressure (mm Hg)?

	Points	
Systolic (top number) BP:	Untreated	Treated with medication
<120	0	0
120–129	1	3
130–139	2	4
140–159	3	5
≥160	4	6

6. What is your 10-year risk?

Points total:	≤9–12	13–14	15	16	17	18	19	20	21	22	23	24	≥25
Ten-year risk percentage:	≤1	2	3	4	5	6	8	11	14	17	22	27	≥30

MY 10-YEAR RISK IS ____________%

Source: Adapted from NCEP, "High Blood Cholesterol, What You Need to Know," available at www.nhlbi.nih.gov/health/public/heart/chol/hbc_what.htm. The 10-Year Heart Attack Risk Calculator can also be accessed on the NHLBI website: www.nhlbi.nih.gov/health/index.htm.

3. Determine Your Risk Category

When you visit your physician, they will complete a more complicated assessment of your risk and look beyond simply your LDL cholesterol value, as high LDL cholesterol is only one major risk factor. Your doctor will likely determine your chances of developing heart disease using the NCEP protocol, a multi-step calculation based on a point system that incorporates LDL in combination with several other risk factors, such as a strong family history of cardiovascular disease and your Framingham ten-year risk score.

Your final score enables your doctor to categorize you into a five-tier risk stratum: Category I, very high risk; Category II, high risk; Category III, moderately high risk; Category IV, moderate risk; and Category V, lower risk. These categories direct and facilitate treatment protocols for physicians to treat patients depending on their level of risk. (Each category has a different LDL goal, with the highest risk, Category I, having the lowest LDL goal number.) Refer to the chart on the next page to calculate your treatment category.

Heart Health on the Internet

For everything you need to know about heart health, plus many delicious heart healthy recipes, please refer to the following websites.

American Heart Association (www.heart.org)
The Centers for Disease Control and Prevention (www.cdc.gov)
The National Heart, Lung, and Blood Institute (www.nhlbi.nih.gov)
Harvard Health Publishing (www.health.harvard.edu)
American Institute for Cancer Research Healthy Recipes (www.aicr.org/cancer-prevention/recipes)

What Is My Treatment Category?

Utilizing your medical history, your number of major risk factors, and 10-year risk score enables your physician to categorize you into a treatment category and give you an LDL goal. Your physician may use this method to determine treatment options for you—and whether you are a potential candidate for statin drug therapy.

Medical History and 10-year Risk Score	Treatment Category	LDL Goal	Possible Treatment Options
Previously diagnosed cardiovascular disease *together with* any of the following: multiple risk factors (especially diabetes), continued smoking, metabolic syndrome, or a recent heart attack	Very high risk	Below 70 mg/dL	Diet and exercise, plus your MD will consider drug treatment
Previously diagnosed cardiovascular disease *or* diabetes *or* 2 or more risk factors that give you a 10-year risk of >20 percent	High risk	Below 100 mg/dL	Diet and exercise, plus your MD will consider drug treatment
2 or more risk factors *and* a 10-year risk of 10–20 percent	Moderately high risk	Below 130 mg/dL	Diet and exercise, plus your MD may consider drug treatment to get LDL to <100 mg/dL

2 or more risk factors *and* a 10-year risk of <10 percent	Moderate risk	Below 130 mg/dL	Diet and exercise, plus your MD may consider drug treatment if LDL ≥160 mg/dL
0–1 risk factors	Lower risk	Below 160 mg/dL	Diet and exercise, plus your MD may consider drug treatment if LDL ≥190 mg/dL or LDL is 160–189 mg/dL *and* 1 severe risk factor
Source: Adapted from Scott M. Grundy et al., "2018 AHA/ACC/AACVPR/AAPA/ABC/ACPM/ADA/AGS/APhA/ASPC/NLA/PCNA Guideline on the Management of Blood Cholesterol: Executive Summary: A Report of the American College of Cardiology/American Heart Association Task Force on Clinical Practice Guidelines," *Journal of the American College of Cardiology* 73, no. 24 (2019): 3168–3209.			

Notes

Foreword

1. Dean Ornish et al., "Intensive Lifestyle Changes for Reversal of Coronary Heart Disease," *JAMA* 280 (1998): 2001–2007.

2. William P. Castelli et al., "Incidence of Coronary Heart Disease and Lipoprotein Cholesterol Levels: The Framingham Study," *JAMA* 256 (1986): 2835–2838; James D. Neaton and Deborah Wentworth, "Serum Cholesterol, Blood Pressure, Cigarette Smoking, and Death from Coronary Heart Disease: Overall Findings and Differences by Age for 316,099 White Men, Multiple Risk Factor Intervention Group," *Archives of Internal Medicine* 152 (1992): 56–64.

3. Donna K. Arnett et al., "2019 ACC/AHA Guideline on the Primary Prevention of Cardiovascular Disease: A Report of the American College of Cardiology/American Heart Association Task Force on Clinical Practice Guidelines," *Circulation* 140, no. 11 (March 17, 2019), https://doi.org/10.1161/cir.0000000000000678.

4. Terje R. Pedersen et al., "Randomised Trial of Cholesterol Lowering in 4444 Patients with Coronary Heart Disease: The Scandinavian Simvastatin Survival Study (4S)," *Lancet* 344 (1994): 1383–1389.

5. B. Mihaylova et al., "The Effects of Lowering LDL Cholesterol With Statin Therapy in People at Low Risk of Vascular Disease: Meta-analysis of Individual Data From 27 Randomised Trials," *The Lancet* 380, no. 9841 (August 1, 2012): 581–90, https://doi.org/10.1016/s0140-6736(12)60367-5.

6. Malin Schoeneck and David Iggman, "The Effects of Foods on LDL Cholesterol Levels: A Systematic Review of the Accumulated Evidence From Systematic Reviews and Meta-analyses of Randomized Controlled Trials," *Nutrition Metabolism and Cardiovascular Diseases* 31, no. 5 (January 18, 2021): 1325–38, https://doi.org/10.1016/j.numecd.2020.12.032.

7. Shufen Han et al., "Effects of Plant Stanol or Sterol-enriched Diets on Lipid Profiles in Patients Treated With Statins: Systematic Review and Meta-analysis," *Scientific Reports* 6, no. 1 (August 19, 2016), https://doi.org/10.1038/srep31337.

8. Donald M. Lloyd-Jones et al., "Life's Essential 8: Updating and Enhancing the American Heart Association's Construct of Cardiovascular Health: A Presidential Advisory From the American Heart Association," *Circulation* 146, no. 5 (June 29, 2022), https://doi.org/10.1161/cir.0000000000001078.

Chapter 1. Cholesterol 101

1. Seth S. Martin et al., "2024 Heart Disease and Stroke Statistics: A Report of US and Global Data From the American Heart Association," *Circulation* 149, no. 8 (January 24, 2024), https://doi.org/10.1161/cir.0000000000001209.
2. Ibid.
3. "Women and Heart Disease," National Heart, Lung, and Blood Institute, https://www.nhlbi.nih.gov/health/coronary-heart-disease/women (accessed October 1, 2024).
4. Shoko Kobayashi, "The Effect of Polyphenols on Hypercholesterolemia through Inhibiting the Transport and Expression of Niemann–Pick C1-Like 1," *International Journal of Molecular Sciences* 20, no. 19 (2019): 4939, https://doi.org/10.3390/ijms20194939.
5. Michael S. Brown and Joseph L. Goldstein, "How LDL Receptors Influence Cholesterol and Atherosclerosis," *Scientific American* 251, no. 5 (November 1984): 58–66.

Chapter 2. Targeting LDL

1. U.S. Department of Health and Human Services, National Institutes of Health, National Heart, Lung, and Blood Institute, "Blood Cholesterol," NIH Publication No. 22-HL-8191, September 2022, www.nhlbi.nih.gov/health/blood-cholesterol; "High Blood Cholesterol—What You Need to Know," NIH Publication No. 05-3290, revised June 2005, www.nhlbi.nih.gov/health/public/heart/chol/hbc_what.htm.
2. Scott M. Grundy et al., "2018 Cholesterol Guideline: Executive Summary, a Report of the American College of Cardiology/American Heart Association Task Force on Clinical Practice Guidelines," Journal of the American College of Cardiology 73 (2019): 3168–3209; National Heart, Lung, and Blood Institute and the National Institutes of Health, "Third Report of the National Cholesterol Education Program (NCEP) Expert Panel on Detection, Evaluation, and Treatment of High Blood Cholesterol in Adults (Adult Treatment Panel III)," NIH Publication No. 02-5215, September 2002, www.nhlbi.nih.gov/guidelines/cholesterol/atp3_rpt.htm (hereafter cited as "Third Report").
3. Alice H. Lichtenstein et al., Coordinating Committee of the National Cholesterol Education Program, "2021 Dietary Guidance to Improve Cardiovascular Health: A Scientific Statement from the American Heart Association," *Circulation* 144 (2021): e472–e487 Alice H. Lichtenstein et al., "2021 Dietary Guidance to Improve Cardiovascular Health: A Scientific Statement from the American Heart Association," *Circulation* 144 (2021): e472–e487.

4. National Cholesterol Education Program (NCEP) Expert Panel on Detection, Evaluation, and Treatment of High Blood Cholesterol in Adults (Adult Treatment Panel III), "Third Report of the National Cholesterol Education Program (NCEP) Expert Panel on Detection, Evaluation, and Treatment of High Blood Cholesterol in Adults (Adult Treatment Panel III) Final Report," *Circulation* 106 (2002): 3143–3421.

5. Neil J. Stone et al., "2013 ACC/AHA Guideline on the Treatment of Blood Cholesterol to Reduce Atherosclerotic Cardiovascular Risk in Adults: A Report of the American College of Cardiology/American Heart Association Task Force on Practice Guidelines," *Journal of The American College of Cardiology* (2013), doi:10.1161/01.cir.0000437738.63853.7a.

6. Michael S. Brown and Joseph L. Goldstein, "How LDL Receptors Influence Cholesterol and Atherosclerosis," *Scientific American* 251, no. 5 (November 1984): 58–66.

7. Sonia Blanco Mejia et al., "A Meta-Analysis of 46 Studies Identified by the FDA Demonstrates that Soy Protein Decreases Circulating LDL and Total Cholesterol Concentrations in Adults," *American Journal of Clinical Nutrition* 149, no. 6 (June 2019): 968–981; Susan M. Potter et al., "Soy Protein and Isoflavones: Their Effects on Blood Lipids and Bone Density in Postmenopausal Women," *American Journal of Clinical Nutrition* 68 (1998) (Suppl.): 1375S–1379S; Jo Ann Baum et al., "Long-Term Intake of Soy Protein Improves Blood Lipid Profiles and Increases Mononuclear Cell Low-Density-Lipoprotein Receptor Messenger RNA in Hypercholesterolemic, Postmenopausal Women," *American Journal of Clinical Nutrition* 68 (1998): 545–551.

8. Malcolm R. Law and Nicholas J. Wald, "An Ecological Study of Serum Cholesterol and Ischaemic Heart Disease between 1950 and 1990," *European Journal of Clinical Nutrition* 48, no. 5 (May 1994): 305–325.

9. Ancel Keys et al., "The Diet and 15-Year Death Rate in the Seven Countries Study," *American Journal of Epidemiology* 124, no. 6 (December 1986): 903–915.

10. Jeremiah Stamler et al., "Relationship of Baseline Serum Cholesterol Levels in 3 Large Cohorts of Younger Men to Long-Term Coronary, Cardiovascular, and All-Cause Mortality and to Longevity," *JAMA* 284, no. 3 (July 19, 2000): 311–318.

11. A. Richey Sharrett et al., "Coronary Heart Disease Prediction from Lipoprotein Cholesterol Levels, Triglycerides, Lipoprotein (a), Apolipoproteins A-I and B, and HDL Density Subfractions: The Atherosclerosis Risk in Communities (ARIC) Study," *Circulation* 104 (2001): 1108–1113.

12. Jonathan C. Cohen et al., "Sequence Variations in PCSK9, Low LDL, and Protection against Coronary Heart Disease," *New England Journal of Medicine* 354 (2006): 1264–1272.

13. Anca Nistor et al., "The Hyperlipidemic Hamster as a Model of Experimental Atherosclerosis," *Atherosclerosis* 68, nos. 1–2 (November 1987): 159–173.

14. Shi Qiang et al., "Arterial Endothelial Dysfunction in Baboons Fed a High-Cholesterol, High-Fat Diet," *American Journal of Clinical Nutrition* 82, no. 4 (2005): 751–759.

15. ALLHAT Collaborative Research Group, "Major Outcomes in Moderately Hypercholesterolemic, Hypertensive Patients Randomized to Pravastatin vs. Usual Care: The Antihypertensive and Lipid-Lowering Treatment to Prevent Heart Attack Trial (ALLHAT-LLT)," *JAMA* 288 (2002): 2998–3007; Peter S. Sever et al., for the ASCOT Investigators, "Prevention of Coronary and Stroke Events with Atorvastatin in Hypertensive Patients Who Have Average or Lower-Than-Average Cholesterol Concentrations, in the Anglo-Scandinavian Cardiac Outcomes Trial—Lipid Lowering Arm (ASCOT-LLA): A Multicentre Randomised Controlled Trial," *Lancet* 361 (2003): 1149–1158; Heart Protection Study Collaborative Group, MRC/BHF, "Heart Protection Study of Cholesterol Lowering with Simvastatin in 20,536 High-Risk Individuals: A Randomised Placebo-Controlled Trial," *Lancet* 360 (2002): 7–22; James Shepherd et al., on behalf of the PROSPER study group, "Pravastatin in Elderly Individuals at Risk of Vascular Disease (PROSPER): A Randomised Controlled Trial," *Lancet* 360 (2002): 1623–1630; Christopher P. Cannon et al., "Intensive versus Moderate Lipid Lowering with Statins after Acute Coronary Syndromes," *New England Journal of Medicine* 350 (2004): 1495–1504.

16. Malcolm R. Law et al., "Quantifying Effect of Statins on Low-Density Lipoprotein Cholesterol, Ischaemic Heart Disease, and Stroke: Systematic Review and Meta-Analysis," *British Medical Journal* 326 (2003): 1423–1429.

17. Steven E. Nissen et al., "Statin Therapy, LDL Cholesterol, C-Reactive Protein, and Coronary Artery Disease," *American Journal of Cardiology* 96, no. 5A (September 5, 2005): 61F–68F.

18. Steven E. Nissen et al., "Effect of Very High-Intensity Statin Therapy on Regression of Coronary Atherosclerosis: The ASTEROID Trial," *JAMA* 295 (2006): 1556–1565.

19. Omar Mhaimeed et al., "The Importance of LDL-C Lowering in Atherosclerotic Cardiovascular Disease Prevention: Lower for Longer Is Better," *American Journal of Preventive Cardiology* 18 (2024).

20. Harold Bays, "Combination Lipid-Altering Drug Therapy with Statins: An Update," slide no. 5, speaker's notes, www.lipidsonline.org/slides/slide01.cfm?tk=33&pg=1.

21. James M. McKenney, "Selecting Successful Lipid-Lowering Treatments," slide no. 10, speaker's notes, www.lipidsonline.org/slides/slide01.cfm?tk=23.

22. Tatjana Rundek et al., "Atorvastatin Decreases the Coenzyme Q10 Level in the Blood of Patients at Risk for Cardiovascular Disease and Stroke," *Archives of Neurology* 61, no. 6 (June 2004): 889–892.

23. Julian M. Whitaker, "Citizen Petition to Amend Regulations for Statin Drugs to Recommend Coenzyme Q10 Supplementation," Docket No. 02P-0244, U.S. Food and Drug Administration, May 24, 2002. Life Extension Editorial Staff, "Dr. Julian M. Whitaker Petitions FDA," *Life Extension Magazine,* August 2002, scientifically reviewed by Dr. Gary Gonzalez, MD, https://www.lifeextension.com/magazine/2002/8/legalnotes.

24. Tine L. Dohlmann et al., "Coenzyme Q10 Supplementation in Statin Treated

Patients: A Double-Blinded Randomized Placebo-Controlled Trial," *Antioxidants* 11, no. 9 (August 29, 2022): 1698.
25. National Heart, Lung, and Blood Institute and the National Institutes of Health, "Third Report of the National Cholesterol Education Program (NCEP) Expert Panel on Detection, Evaluation, and Treatment of High Blood Cholesterol in Adults (Adult Treatment Panel III)," NIH Publication No. 02-5215, September 2002, www.nhlbi.nih.gov/guidelines/cholesterol/atp3_rpt.htm.

Chapter 3. Cholesterol Down: A Combination Therapy as Effective as Statins

1. David J. A. Jenkins et al., "Direct Comparison of a Dietary Portfolio of Cholesterol-Lowering Foods with a Statin in Hypercholesterolemic Participants," *American Journal of Clinical Nutrition* 81, no. 2 (February 2005): 380–387.
2. David J. A. Jenkins et al., "A Dietary Portfolio Approach to Cholesterol Reduction: Combined Effects of Plant Sterols, Vegetable Proteins, and Viscous Fibers in Hypercholesterolemia," *Metabolism* 51, no. 12 (December 2002): 1596–1604.
3. Kevin C. Maki et al., "Food Products Containing Free Tall Oil–Based Phytosterols and Oat β-Glucan Lower Serum Total and LDL Cholesterol in Hypercholesterolemic Adults," *Journal of Nutrition* 133 (2003): 808–813.
4. Christopher D. Gardner et al., "The Effect of a Plant-Based Diet on Plasma Lipids in Hypercholesterolemic Adults: A Randomized Trial," *Annals of Internal Medicine* 142 (2005): 725–733.
5. Stephen L. Kopecky et al., "Reduction in Serum LDL Cholesterol Using a Nutrient Compendium in Hyperlipidemic Adults Unable or Unwilling to Use Statin Therapy: A Double-Blind Randomized Crossover Clinical Trial," *Journal of Nutrition* 152 (2022): 458–465.
6. Oscar H. Franco et al., "The Polymeal: A Natural, Safer, and Probably Tastier (than the Polypill) Strategy to Reduce Cardiovascular Disease by More than 75%," *British Medical Journal* 329 (December 2004): 1447–1450.
7. The amounts of the food ingredients of the Cholesterol Down Plan specified in each daily prescription are derived from scientific research, NCEP, and the American Heart Association 2000 dietary recommendations. See "Executive Summary of the Third Report of the National Cholesterol Education Program (NCEP) Expert Panel on Detection, Evaluation, and Treatment of High Blood Cholesterol in Adults (Adult Treatment Panel III)," *JAMA* 285 (2001): 2486–2497; Ronald M. Krauss et al., "American Heart Association Dietary Guidelines Revision 2000: A Statement for the Healthcare Professionals from the Nutrition Committee of the American Heart Association," *Circulation* 102 (2000): 2296–2311; Jenkins et al., "Dietary Portfolio Approach to Cholesterol Reduction"; Gardner et al., "Effect of a Plant-Based Diet on Plasma Lipids in Hypercholesterolemic Adults"; Krista A. Varady et al., "Plant Sterols and Endurance Training Combine to Favorably Alter Plasma Lipid Profiles in Previously Sedentary Hypercholesterolemic Adults after 8 Weeks," *American Journal of Clinical Nutrition* 80 (2004): 1159–1166.

Chapter 4. Step 1: Eat Oatmeal

1. David R. Jacobs Jr. et al., "Whole-Grain Intake May Reduce the Risk of Ischemic Heart Disease Death in Postmenopausal Women: The Iowa Women's Health Study," *American Journal of Clinical Nutrition* 68 (1998): 248–257.

2. Umed A. Ajani et al., "Dietary Fiber and C-Reactive Protein: Findings from National Health and Nutrition Examination Survey Data," *Journal of Nutrition* 134 (2004): 1181–1185.

3. Simin Liu et al., "Whole Grain Consumption and Risk of Ischemic Stroke in Women: A Prospective Study," *JAMA* 284, no. 12 (September 27, 2000): 1534–1540.

4. Simin Liu et al., "Is Intake of Breakfast Cereals Related to Total and Cause-Specific Mortality in Men?" *American Journal of Clinical Nutrition* 77 (2003): 594–599.

5. Frank Thies et al., "Oats and Cholesterol: A Systematic Literature Review," *British Journal of Nutrition* 112, no. S2 (October 2014): S19–S30.

6. Ann L. Gerhardt and Noreen B. Gallo, "Full-Fat Rice Bran and Oat Bran Similarly Reduce Hypercholesterolemia in Humans," *Journal of Nutrition* 128 (1998): 865–869.

7. Brenda M. Davy et al., "High-Fiber Oat Cereal Compared with Wheat Cereal Consumption Favorably Alters LDL-Cholesterol Subclass and Particle Numbers in Middle-Aged and Older Men," *American Journal of Clinical Nutrition* 76 (2002): 351–358.

8. Junhui Yu et al., "Effects of Oat Beta-Glucan Intake on Lipid Profiles in Hypercholesterolemic Adults: A Systematic Review and Meta-Analysis of Randomized Controlled Trials," *Nutrients* 14 (2022), https://doi.org/10.3390/nu14102043.

9. Scott M. Grundy et al., "Interruption of the Enterohepatic Circulation of Bile Acids in Man: Comparative Effects of Cholestyramine and Ileal Exclusion on Cholesterol Metabolism," *Journal of Laboratory Clinical Medicine* 78 (1971): 94–121.

10. Michael H. Davidson et al., "The Hypocholesterolemic Effects of Beta-Glucan in Oatmeal and Oat Bran: A Dose-Controlled Study," *JAMA* 265 (1991): 1833–1839.

11. American Heart Association, "Whole Grains, Refined Grains, and Dietary Fiber," last modified November 2024, www.heart.org/en/healthy-living/healthy-eating/eat-smart/nutrition-basics/whole-grains-refined-grains-and-dietary-fiber.

12. Cynthia M. Ripsin et al., "Oat Products and Lipid-Lowering: A Meta-Analysis," *JAMA* 267 (1992): 3317–3325.

13. Chung-Yen Chen et al., "Aventhramides and Phenolic Acids from Oats Are Bioavailable and Act Synergistically with Vitamin C to Enhance Hamster and Human LDL Resistance to Oxidation," *Journal of Nutrition* 134 (2004): 1459–1466.

14. Liping Liu et al., "The Antiatherogenic Potential of Oat Phenolic Compounds," *Atherosclerosis* 175, no. 1 (July 2004): 39–49.

15. Elzbeita M. Kurowska and Kenneth K. Carroll, "LDL versus Apolipoprotein B Responses to Variable Proportions of Selected Amino Acids in Semipurified Diets Fed to Rabbits and in the Media of HepG2 Cells," *Journal of Nutritional Biochemistry* 7 (1996): 418–424.

16. FDA talk paper, "FDA Allows Whole Oat Foods to Make Health Claim on Reducing the Risk of Heart Disease," January 21, 1997, www.cfsan.fda.gov/~lrd/tpoats.html.

Chapter 5. Step 2: Eat Almonds

1. Gary E. Fraser, "Nut Consumption, Lipids, and Risk of a Coronary Event," *Clinical Cardiology* 22 (July 1999) (Suppl. III): III-11–III-15.
2. Gary E. Fraser et al., "A Possible Protective Effect of Nut Consumption on Risk of Coronary Heart Disease: The Adventist Health Study," *Archives of Internal Medicine* 152 (1992): 1416–1424.
3. Soumik Kalita et al., "Almonds and Cardiovascular Health: A Review," *Nutrients* 10 (2018): 468, doi:10.3390/nu10040468.
4. Mavis Abbey et al., "Partial Replacement of Saturated Fatty Acids with Almonds or Walnuts Lowers Total Plasma Cholesterol and Low-Density-Lipoprotein Cholesterol," *American Journal of Clinical Nutrition* 59 (1994): 995–999.
5. Joan Sabaté et al., "Serum Lipid Response to the Graduated Enrichment of a Step 1 Diet with Almonds: A Randomized Feeding Trial," *American Journal of Clinical Nutrition* 77 (2003): 1379–1384.
6. Gene A. Spiller et al., "Effects of Plant-Based Diets High in Raw or Roasted Almonds, or Roasted Almond Butter on Serum Lipoproteins in Humans," *Journal of the American College of Nutrition* 22, no. 3 (2003): 195–200.
7. Gene A. Spiller et al., "Nuts and Plasma Lipids: An Almond-Based Diet Lowers LDL-C while Preserving HDL-C," *Journal of the American College of Nutrition* 17, no. 3 (1998): 285–290.
8. James W. Anderson et al., "Health Benefits and Practical Aspects of High-Fiber Diets," *American Journal of Clinical Nutrition* 59, no. 5 (1994 Suppl.): 1242S–1247S.
9. Rachel R. Huxley and H. Andrew Neil, "The Relation Between Dietary Flavonol Intake and Coronary Heart Disease Mortality: A Meta-Analysis of Prospective Cohort Studies," *European Journal of Clinical Nutrition* 57 (2003): 904–908.
10. Bianca Fuhrman and Michael Aviram, "Flavonoids Protect LDL from Oxidation and Attenuate Atherosclerosis," *Current Opinions in Lipidology* 12 (2001): 41–48.
11. Chung-Yen Chen et al., "Flavonoids from Almond Skins Are Bioavailable and Act Synergistically with Vitamins C and E to Enhance Hamster and Human LDL Resistance to Oxidation," *Journal of Nutrition* 135 (2005): 1366–1373.
12. Frank M. Sacks and Hannia Campos, "Low-Density Lipoprotein Size and Cardiovascular Disease: A Reappraisal," *Journal of Clinical Endocrinology and Metabolism* 88, no. 10 (2003): 4525–4532.
13. Edgar R. Miller III et al., "Meta-Analysis: High-Dosage Vitamin E Supplementation May Increase All-Cause Mortality," *Annals of Internal Medicine* 142 (January 2005): 37–46.
14. MRC/BHF Heart Protection Study Collaborative Group, "MRC/BHF Heart

Protection Study of Antioxidant Vitamin Supplementation in 20,536 High-Risk Individuals: A Randomized Placebo-Controlled Trial," *Lancet* 360 (July 6, 2002): 23–33.
15. Laura A. Yochum et al., "Intake of Antioxidant Vitamins and Risk of Death from Stroke in Postmenopausal Women," *American Journal of Clinical Nutrition* 72, no. 2 (August 2000): 476–483.
16. Office of Dietary Supplements, "Health Professional Fact Sheet on Vitamin E," National Institutes of Health, https://ods.od.nih.gov/factsheets.

Chapter 6. Step 3: Eat Flaxseeds

1. Wioletta Nowak and Małgorzata Jeziorek, "The Role of Flaxseed in Improving Human Health," *Healthcare* 11, no. 3 (January 30, 2023): 395, doi:10.3390/healthcare11030395.
2. Esther Lopez-Garcia et al., "Consumption of (N-3) Fatty Acids Is Related to Plasma Biomarkers of Inflammation and Endothelial Activation in Women," *Journal of Nutrition* 134 (2004): 1806–1811.
3. Guixiang Zhao et al., "Dietary α-Linolenic Acid Reduces Inflammatory and Lipid Cardiovascular Risk Factors in Hypercholesterolemic Men and Women," *Journal of Nutrition* 134 (2004): 2991–2997.
4. Tetsuro Yamashita et al., "Varying the Ratio of Dietary N-6/N-3 Polyunsaturated Fatty Acids Alters the Tendency to Thrombosis and Progression of Atherosclerosis in ApoE (-/-) LDLR (-/-) Double Knockout Mouse," *Thrombosis Research* 116, no. 5 (2005): 393–401.
5. Brenda C. Davis and Penny M. Kris-Etherton, "Achieving Optimal Essential Fatty Acid Status in Vegetarians: Current Knowledge and Practical Applications," *American Journal of Clinical Nutrition* 78 (Suppl.) (2003): 640S–646S.
6. LeAnne T. Bloedon and Philippe O. Szapary, "Flaxseed and Cardiovascular Risk," *Nutrition Reviews* 62, no. 1 (2004): 18–27; Edralin A. Lucas et al., "Flaxseed Improves Lipid Profile Without Altering Biomarkers of Bone Metabolism in Postmenopausal Women," *Journal of Clinical Endocrinology and Metabolism* 87, no. 4 (April 2002): 1527–1532; Leisa Ridges et al., "Cholesterol Lowering Benefits of Soy and Linseed Enriched Foods," *Asia Pacific Journal of Clinical Nutrition* 10, no. 3 (2001): 204–211; Marvin L. Bierenbaum et al., "Reducing Atherogenic Risk in Hyperlipemic Humans with Flax Seed Supplementation: A Preliminary Report," *Journal of the American College of Nutrition* 12, no. 5 (October 1993): 501–504.
7. Bahram H. Arjmandi et al., "Whole Flaxseed Consumption Lowers Serum LDL-Cholesterol and Lipoprotein (A) Concentrations in Postmenopausal Women," *Nutrition Research* 18, no. 7 (July 1998): 1203–1214.
8. David J. A. Jenkins et al., "Health Aspects of Partially Defatted Flaxseed, Including Effects on Serum Lipids, Oxidative Measures, and Ex Vivo Androgen and Progestin Activity: A Controlled Crossover Trial," *American Journal of Clinical Nutrition* 69 (1999): 395–402.
9. Kailash Prasad, "Reduction of Serum Cholesterol and Hypercholesterolemic

Atherosclerosis in Rabbits by Secoisolariciresinol Diglucoside Isolated from Flaxseed," *Circulation* 99 (1999): 1355–1362.
10. Lucas et al., "Flaxseed Improves Lipid Profile."
11. Hong Shen et al., "Dietary Soluble Fiber Lowers Plasma LDL Cholesterol Concentrations by Altering Lipoprotein Metabolism in Female Guinea Pigs," *Journal of Nutrition* 128 (1998): 1434–1441.
12. Paul Kuo et al., "Plasma Membrane Enrichment with Cis-Unsaturated Fatty Acids Enhances LDL Metabolism in U937 Monocytes," *Arteriosclerosis* 10 (January/February 1990): 111–118.

Chapter 7. Step 4: Take a Psyllium Fiber Supplement

1. Zhang et al., "Association Between Dietary Fiber Intake and Atherosclerotic Cardiovascular Disease Risk in Adults: A Cross-Sectional Study of 14,947 Population Based on the National Health and Nutrition Examination Surveys," BMC Public Health 22 (2022), https://doi.org/10.1186/s12889-022-13419-y.
2. Mark A. Pereira et al., "Dietary Fiber and Risk of Coronary Heart Disease: A Pooled Analysis of Cohort Studies," Archives of Internal Medicine 164, no. 4 (February 23, 2004): 370–376.
3. Ruth Papazian, "Bulking Up Fiber's Healthful Reputation; More Benefits of Roughage Are Discovered," U.S. Food and Drug Administration, www.fda.gov/fdac/features/1997/597_fiber.html.
4. David J. A. Jenkins et al., "Viscous Fibers, Health Claims, and Strategies to Reduce Cardiovascular Disease Risk," *American Journal of Clinical Nutrition* 71 (2000): 401–402.
5. Alexandra L. Jenkins et al., "Fiber in the Treatment of Hyperlipidemia," in *CRC Handbook of Dietary Fiber in Human Nutrition*, 3rd ed., ed. Gene A. Spiller (Boca Raton, Fla.: CRC Press, 2001), 401–421.
6. Judith A. Marlett et al., "An Unfermented Gel Component of Psyllium Seed Husk Promotes Laxation as a Lubricant in Humans," *American Journal of Clinical Nutrition* 72 (2000): 784–789.
7. Ana Lourdes Romero et al., "Cookies Enriched with Psyllium or Oat Bran Lower Plasma LDL Cholesterol in Normal and Hypercholesterolemic Men from Northern Mexico," *Journal of the American College of Nutrition* 17, no. 6 (1998): 601–608.
8. James W. Anderson et al., "Cholesterol-Lowering Effects of Psyllium Hydrophilic Mucilloid for Hypercholesterolemic Men," *Archives of Internal Medicine* 148, no. 2 (1988): 292–296, doi:10.1001/archinte.1988.00380020036007.
9. James W. Anderson et al., "Cholesterol-Lowering Effects of Psyllium-Enriched Cereal as an Adjunct to a Prudent Diet in the Treatment of Mild to Moderate Hypercholesterolemia," *American Journal of Clinical Nutrition* 56 (1992): 93–98.
10. Beth H. Olson et al., "Psyllium-Enriched Cereals Lower Blood Total Cholesterol and LDL Cholesterol, but Not HDL Cholesterol, in Hypercholesterolemic Adults: Results of a Meta-Analysis," *Journal of Nutrition* 127 (1997): 1973–1980.

11. Marcela Vergara-Jiminez et al., "Hypolipidemic Mechanisms of Pectin and Psyllium in Guinea Pigs Fed High Fat-Sucrose Diets: Alterations on Hepatic Cholesterol Metabolism," *Journal of Lipid Research* 39 (1998): 1455–1465.
12. Ibid.

Chapter 8. Step 5: Eat Beans

1. Pramil N. Singh et al., "Does Low Meat Consumption Increase Life Expectancy in Humans?" *American Journal of Clinical Nutrition* 78 (Suppl.) (2003): 526S–532S; Irene Darmadi-Blackberry et al., "Legumes: The Most Important Dietary Predictor of Survival in Older People of Different Ethnicities," *Asia Pacific Journal of Clinical Nutrition* 13, no. 2 (2004): 217–220.
2. Lydia A. Bazzano et al., "Legume Consumption and Risk of Coronary Heart Disease in US Men and Women," *Archives of Internal Medicine* 161 (2001): 2573–2578.
3. James W. Anderson et al., "Hypocholesterolemic Effects of Oat-Bran or Bean Intake for Hypercholesterolemic Men," *American Journal of Clinical Nutrition* 40, no. 6 (December 1984): 1146–1155.
4. James W. Anderson and Amy W. Major, "Pulses and Lipaemia, Short- and Long-Term Effect: Potential in the Prevention of Cardiovascular Disease," *British Journal of Nutrition* 88 (Suppl. 3) (December 2002): S263–S271.
5. Katarina M. Doma et al., "Canned Beans Decrease Serum Total and LDL Cholesterol in Adults with Elevated LDL Cholesterol in a 4-Wk Multicenter, Randomized, Crossover Study," *Journal of Nutrition* 151 (2021): 3701–3709.
6. James W. Anderson et al., "Cardiovascular and Renal Benefits of Dry Bean and Soybean Intake," *American Journal of Clinical Nutrition* 70 (1999) (Suppl.): S464–S474.
7. Marcela Vergara-Jiminez et al., "Hypolipidemic Mechanisms of Pectin and Psyllium in Guinea Pigs Fed High Fat-Sucrose Diets: Alterations on Hepatic Cholesterol Metabolism," *Journal of Lipid Research* 39 (1998): 1455–1465.

Chapter 9. Step 6: Eat Apples

1. Hong Shen et al., "Dietary Soluble Fiber Lowers Plasma LDL Cholesterol Concentrations by Altering Lipoprotein Metabolism in Female Guinea Pigs," *Journal of Nutrition* 128 (1998): 1434–1441.
2. Marcela Vergara-Jiminez et al., "Hypolipidemic Mechanisms of Pectin and Psyllium in Guinea Pigs Fed High Fat-Sucrose Diets: Alterations on Hepatic Cholesterol Metabolism," *Journal of Lipid Research* 39 (1998): 1455–1465.
3. Huiyun Wu et al., "Dietary Fiber and Progression of Atherosclerosis: The Los Angeles Atherosclerosis Study," *American Journal of Clinical Nutrition* 78 (2003): 1085–1091.
4. Gian Carlo Tenore et al., "Annurca (Malus pumila Miller cv. Annurca) Apple as a Functional Food for the Contribution to a Healthy Balance of Plasma Cholesterol

Levels: Results of a Randomized Clinical Trial," *Journal of the Science of Food and Agriculture* 97, no. 7 (May 2017): 2107–2115, doi:10.1002/jsfa.8016.
5. Deborah A. Pearson et al., "Apple Juice Inhibits Human Low-Density Lipoprotein Oxidation," *Life Sciences* 64, no. 21 (1999): 1913–1920.
6. Yi-Fang Chu and Rui Hai Liu, "Apple Phytochemicals Inhibit Human LDL Oxidation and Induce LDL Receptor Expression in Hepatocytes," paper presented at the Graduate Student Symposium, Division of Agricultural and Food Chemistry, 229th ACS National Meeting, San Diego, California, March 13–17, 2005.
7. Oliver Aprikian et al., "Lyophilized Apple Counteracts the Development of Hypercholesterolemia, Oxidative Stress, and Renal Dysfunction in Obese Zucker Rats," *Journal of Nutrition* 132 (2002): 1969–1976.
8. Oliver Aprikian et al., "Apple Pectin and a Polyphenol-Rich Apple Concentrate Are More Effective Together than Separately on Cecal Fermentations and Plasma Lipids in Rats," *Journal of Nutrition* 133 (2003): 1860–1865.
9. Tosca L. Zern and Maria Luz Fernandez, "Cardioprotective Effects of Dietary Polyphenols," *Journal of Nutrition* 135 (2005): 2291–2294.
10. Tosca L. Zern et al., "Grape Polyphenols Exert a Cardioprotective Effect in Pre- and Postmenopausal Women by Lowering Plasma Lipids and Reducing Oxidative Stress," *Journal of Nutrition* 135 (2005): 1911–1917.
11. Walter J. Krol et al., "Reduction of Pesticide Residues on Produce by Rinsing," *Journal of Agriculture and Food Chemistry* 48 (2000): 4666–4670.

Chapter 10. Step 7: Take Phytosterols

1. Fotios Barkas et al., "Plant Sterols and Plant Stanols in Cholesterol Management and Cardiovascular Prevention," *Nutrients* 15, no. 13 (2023), https://doi.org/10.3390/nu15132845.
2. National Heart, Lung, and Blood Institute and the National Institutes of Health, "Third Report of the National Cholesterol Education Program (NCEP) Expert Panel on Detection, Evaluation, and Treatment of High Blood Cholesterol in Adults (Adult Treatment Panel III)," NIH Publication No. 02-5215, September 2002, V-14, www.nhlbi.nih.gov/guidelines/cholesterol/atp3_rpt.htm.
3. O. J. Pollack, "Reduction of Blood Cholesterol in Man," *Circulation* 7 (1953): 702–706.
4. Tatu A. Miettinen et al., "Reduction of Serum Cholesterol with Sitostanol-Ester Margarine in a Mildly Hypercholesteremic Population," *New England Journal of Medicine* 333 (1995): 1308–1312.
5. Maarit A. Hallikainen et al., "Comparison of the Effects of Plant Sterol Ester and Plant Stanol Ester-Enriched Margarines in Lowering Serum Cholesterol Concentrations in Hypercholesterolaemic Subjects on a Low-Fat Diet," *European Journal of Clinical Nutrition* 54, no. 9 (September 2000): 715–725.
6. Kevin C. Maki et al., "Lipid Responses to Plant-Sterol-Enriched Reduced-Fat Spreads Incorporated into a National Cholesterol Education Program Step 1 Diet," *American Journal of Clinical Nutrition* 74 (2001): 33–43.

7. "FDA Authorizes New Coronary Heart Disease Health Claim for Plant Sterol and Plant Stanol Esters," talk paper, U.S. Food and Drug Administration, September 5, 2000, www.cfsan.fda.gov/~lrd/tpsterol.html.
8. A. Poli et al., "Phytosterols, Cholesterol Control, and Cardiovascular Disease," *Nutrients* 13, no. 8 (2021): 2810, https://doi.org/10.3390/nu13082810.
9. National Heart, Lung, and Blood Institute and the National Institutes of Health, "Third Report of the National Cholesterol Education Program (NCEP) Expert Panel on Detection, Evaluation, and Treatment of High Blood Cholesterol in Adults (Adult Treatment Panel III)."
10. Suhad S. AbuMweis et al., "Intake of a Single Morning Dose of Standard and Novel Plant Sterol Preparations for 4 Weeks Does Not Dramatically Affect Plasma Lipid Concentrations in Humans," *Journal of Nutrition* 136 (2006): 1012–1016.
11. Manny Noakes et al., "An Increase in Dietary Carotenoids When Consuming Plant Sterols or Stanols Is Effective in Maintaining Plasma Carotenoid Concentrations," *American Journal of Clinical Nutrition* 75 (2002): 79–86.

Chapter 11. Step 8: Eat Soy Protein

1. James W. Anderson et al., "Meta-Analysis of the Effects of Soy Protein Intake on Serum Lipids," *New England Journal of Medicine* 333 (August 1995): 276–282.
2. Sonia Blanco Mejia et al., "A Meta-Analysis of 46 Studies Identified by the FDA Demonstrates that Soy Protein Decreases Circulating LDL and Total Cholesterol Concentrations in Adults," *Journal of Nutrition* 149 (2019): 968–981.
3. Xing-Gang Zhuo et al., "Soy Isoflavone Intake Lowers Serum LDL Cholesterol: A Meta-Analysis of 8 Randomized Controlled Trials in Humans," *Journal of Nutrition* 134 (September 2004): 2395–2400.
4. Daniëlle A. J. M. Kerckhoffs et al., "Effects on the Human Serum Lipoprotein Profile of β-Glucan, Soy Protein and Isoflavones, Plant Sterols and Stanols, Garlic, and Tocotrienols," *Journal of Nutrition* 132 (2002): 2494–2505.
5. Sophie Desroches et al., "Soy Protein Favorably Affects LDL Size Independently of Isoflavones in Hypercholesterolemic Men and Women," *Journal of Nutrition* 134 (March 2004): 574–579.
6. U.S. Food and Drug Administration, "Food Labeling: Health Claims; Soy Protein and Coronary Heart Disease," final rule, *Federal Register* 64 (1999): 57700–57733; "New Health Claim Proposed for Relationship of Soy Protein and Coronary Heart Disease," talk paper, U.S. Food and Drug Administration, November 10, 1998.
7. M. R. Lovati et al., "Soybean Protein Diet Increases Low Density Lipoprotein Receptor Activity in Mononuclear Cells from Hypercholesterolemic Patients," *Journal of Clinical Investigation* 80 (1987): 1498–1502.
8. Michael R. Adams et al., "Dietary Soy β-Conglycinin (7S Globulin) Inhibits Atherosclerosis in Mice," *Journal of Nutrition* 134 (2004): 511–516.
9. Marcello Duranti et al., "The α Subunit from Soybean 7S Globulin Lowers Plasma Lipids and Upregulates Liver β-VLDL Receptors in Rats Fed a Hypercholesterolemic Diet," *Journal of Nutrition* 134 (2004): 1334–1339.

10. Elzbieta M. Kurowska and Kenneth K. Carroll, "LDL versus Apolipoprotein B Responses to Variable Proportions of Selected Amino Acids in Semipurified Diets Fed to Rabbits and in the Media HepG2 Cells," *Journal of Nutritional Biochemistry* 7 (1996): 418–424.

Chapter 12. Step 9: Eat Fewer Calories

1. K. M. Huffman et al., "Calorie Restriction Improves Lipid-Related Emerging Cardiometabolic Risk Factors in Healthy Adults without Obesity: Distinct Influences of BMI and Sex from CALERIE a Multicentre, Phase 2, Randomized Controlled Trial," *eClinicalMedicine,* January 3, 2022, https://doi.org/10.1016/j.eclinm.2021.101261.

2. R. J. Henning, "Obesity and Obesity-Induced Inflammatory Disease Contribute to Atherosclerosis: A Review of the Pathophysiology and Treatment of Obesity," *American Journal of Cardiovascular Disease* 11, no. 4 (2021): 504–529.

3. X. Zhang et al., "Body Roundness Index and All-Cause Mortality Among US Adults," *JAMA Network Open* 7, no. 6 (June 5, 2024): e2415051, doi: 10.1001/jamanetworkopen.2024.15051.

4. M. Bo et al., "Body Fat and C-Reactive Protein Levels in Healthy Non-Obese Men," *Nutrition, Metabolism, and Cardiovascular Diseases* 14, no. 2 (April 2004): 66–72.

5. Z. Ungvari et al., "Mechanisms Underlying Caloric Restriction and Lifespan Regulation: Implications for Vascular Aging," *Circulation* 102, no. 5 (March 14, 2008): 519–528.

6. The Diabetes Prevention Program Research Group, "Reduction in the Incidence of Type 2 Diabetes with Lifestyle Intervention or Metformin," *New England Journal of Medicine* 346 (2002): 393–403.

7. Welton S., Minty R., O'Driscoll T., et al., "Intermittent fasting and weight loss systematic review," *Canadian Family Physician* 66 (2020): 117–125.

8. S. Keenan et al., "The Effects of Intermittent Fasting and Continuous Energy Restriction with Exercise on Cardiometabolic Biomarkers, Dietary Compliance, and Perceived Hunger and Mood: Secondary Outcomes of a Randomised, Controlled Trial," *Nutrients* 14 (2022): 2–18.

9. S. Welton et al., "Intermittent Fasting and Weight Loss Systematic Review," *Canadian Family Physician* 66 (2020): 117–125.

10. National Restaurant Association, "State of the Restaurant Industry Report," 2024, https://restaurant.org/research-and-media/research/industry-statistics/state-of-the-industry/.

11. Lorien E. Urban et al., "The Energy Content of Restaurant Foods Without Stated Calorie Information," *JAMA Internal Medicine* 173, no. 14 (2013): 1292–1299.

12. S. Keenan et al., "The Effects of Intermittent Fasting and Continuous Energy Restriction with Exercise on Cardiometabolic Biomarkers, Dietary Compliance, and Perceived Hunger and Mood: Secondary Outcomes of a Randomised, Controlled Trial," *Nutrients* 14 (2022): 2–18.

Chapter 13. Step 10: Walk

1. P. C. Dempsey et al., "Investigation of a UK Biobank Cohort Reveals Causal Associations of Self-Reported Walking Pace with Telomere Length," *Communications Biology* 5 (2022), doi:10.1038/s42003-022-03323-x.
2. Nazik Elgaddal et al., "Physical Activity Among Adults Aged 18 and Over: United States, 2020," *NCHS DATA BRIEF* no. 433 (2022), https://dx.doi.org/10.15620/cdc:120213.
3. Kosuke Inoue et al., "Association of Daily Step Patterns With Mortality in US Adults," *JAMA Network Open* 6, no. 3 (2023): e235174.
4. George A. Kelley et al., "Walking, Lipids, and Lipoproteins: A Meta-Analysis of Randomized Controlled Trials," *Preventive Medicine* 38, no. 5 (May 2004): 651–661.
5. American Heart Association, *Heart Disease and Stroke Statistics—2006 Update* (Dallas: American Heart Association, 2006).
6. Andrea Kriska, "Can a Physically Active Lifestyle Prevent Type 2 Diabetes?" *Exercise and Sports Sciences Reviews* 31, no. 3 (July 2003): 132–137.
7. Oscar H. Franco et al., "Effects of Physical Activity on Life Expectancy with Cardiovascular Disease," *Archives of Internal Medicine* 165, no. 20 (November 14, 2005): 2355–2360.
8. Alpa V. Patel et al., "Lifetime Recreational Exercise Activity and Risk of Breast Carcinoma in Situ," *Cancer* 98 (2003): 2161–2169; Michelle D. Holmes et al., "Physical Activity and Survival After Breast Cancer Diagnosis," *JAMA* 293, no. 20 (May 25, 2005): 2479–2486; A. K. A. Samad et al., "A Meta-Analysis of the Association of Physical Activity with Reduced Risk of Colorectal Cancer," *Colorectal Disease* 7, no. 3 (May 2005): 204–213.
9. Jerome L. Fleg et al., "Accelerated Longitudinal Decline of Aerobic Capacity in Healthy Older Adults," *Circulation* 112 (2005): 674–682.
10. Suvi Rovio et al., "Leisure-Time Physical Activity at Midlife and the Risk of Dementia and Alzheimer's Disease," *Lancet Neurology* 4, no. 11 (November 2005): 705–711.
11. Tedd L. Mitchell et al., "Effects of Cardiorespiratory Fitness on Healthcare Utilization," *Medicine and Science in Sports and Exercise* 36, no. 12 (2004): 2088–2092.
12. Expert Panel on Detection, Evaluation, and Treatment of High Blood Cholesterol in Adults, "Executive Summary of the Third Report of the National Cholesterol Education Program (NCEP) Expert Panel on Detection, Evaluation, and Treatment of High Blood Cholesterol in Adults (Adult Treatment Panel III)," *JAMA* 285 (2001): 2486–2497.
13. Zung Vu Tran and Arthur Weltman, "Differential Effects of Exercise on Serum Lipid and Lipoprotein Levels Seen with Changes in Body Weight," *JAMA* 254, no. 7 (August 16, 1985): 919–924.
14. Kelley et al., "Walking, Lipids, and Lipoproteins."
15. Amy A. Hakim et al., "Effects of Walking on Mortality among Nonsmoking Retired Men," *New England Journal of Medicine* 338 (1998): 94–99.

16. Gang Hu et al., "Leisure Time, Occupational, and Commuting Physical Activity and the Risk of Stroke," *Stroke* 36 (2005): 1994–1999.
17. Marcia L. Stefanick et al., "Effects of Diet and Exercise in Men and Postmenopausal Women with Low Levels of HDL Cholesterol and High Levels of LDL Cholesterol," *New England Journal of Medicine* 339 (July 2, 1998): 12–20.
18. Stefano Sdringola et al., "Combined Intense Lifestyle and Pharmacologic Lipid Treatment Further Reduce Coronary Events and Myocardial Perfusion Abnormalities Compared with Usual-Care Cholesterol-Lowering Drugs in Coronary Artery Disease," *Journal of the American College of Cardiology* 41, no. 2 (2003): 263–272.
19. Jose Luis Sánchez-Quesada et al., "LDL from Aerobically Trained Subjects Shows Higher Resistance to Oxidative Modification than LDL from Sedentary Subjects," *Atherosclerosis* 132, no. 2 (July 25, 1997): 207–213.
20. Tommi J. Vasankari et al., "Reduced Oxidized LDL Levels After a 10-Month Exercise Program," *Medicine and Science in Sports and Exercise* 30, no. 10 (October 1998): 1496–1501.
21. Nobushige Yamashita et al., "Exercise Provides Direct Biphasic Cardioprotection via Manganese Superoxide Dismutase Activation," *Journal of Experimental Medicine* 189, no. 11 (June 7, 1999): 1699–1706.
22. William E. Kraus et al., "Effects of the Amount and Intensity of Exercise on Plasma Lipoproteins," *New England Journal of Medicine* 347, no. 19 (November 7, 2002): 1483–1492.
23. Mark A. Sarzynski et al., "The Effects of Exercise on the Lipoprotein Subclass Profile: A Meta-Analysis of 10 Interventions," *Atherosclerosis* 243, no. 2 (December 2015): 364–372.
24. Alan R. Tall, "Exercise to Reduce Cardiovascular Risk—How Much Is Enough?" *New England Journal of Medicine* 347, no. 19 (November 7, 2002): 1522–1524.
25. Jean-Pierre Després et al., "Long-Term Exercise Training with Constant Energy Intake. 3. Effects on Plasma Lipoprotein Levels," *International Journal of Obesity* 14, no. 1 (1990): 85–94.
26. Julie Y. Ji et al., "Shear Stress Causes Nuclear Localization of Endothelial Glucocorticoid Receptor and Expression from the GRE Promoter," *Circulation Research* 92 (2003): 279–285.
27. Adel M. Malek et al., "Hemodynamic Shear Stress and Its Role in Atherosclerosis," *JAMA* 282 (1999): 2035–2042.
28. J. Kelly Smith et al., "Long-Term Exercise and Atherogenic Activity of Blood Mononuclear Cells in Persons at Risk of Developing Ischemic Heart Disease," *JAMA* 281, no. 18 (1999): 1722–1727.

A Few Closing Words from Dr. Janet

1. Omar Mhaimeed et al., "The Importance of LDL-C Lowering in Atherosclerotic Cardiovascular Disease Prevention: Lower for Longer Is Better," *American Journal of Preventive Cardiology* 18 (2024): 100649.

2. Alan R. Tall, "Protease Variants, LDL, and Coronary Heart Disease," *New England Journal of Medicine* 354, no. 12 (2006): 1310–1312.

Appendix 5. What's Your Risk of Heart Disease?

1. William B. Kannel et al., "Factors of Risk in the Development of Coronary Heart Disease—Six-Year Follow-Up Experience; the Framingham Study," *Annals of Internal Medicine* 55 (1961): 33–50.
2. Philip Greenland et al., "Major Risk Factors as Antecedents of Fatal and Nonfatal Coronary Heart Disease Events," *JAMA* 290, no. 7 (2003): 891–897.

Acknowledgments

I am deeply grateful to the many people who contributed to the completion of this book. I would like to begin by expressing my heartfelt thanks to my literary agent, Faith Hamlin, who took a chance on a novice author and gave me the opportunity I could only have imagined in my dreams. Thank you, Faith, for everything. You are kind, you are encouraging, you are my friend, and you are the best at what you do.

I owe everything to my mother, Dr. Alma Bond, who passed away in 2021. She was a much-published author who in my initial writing of this book helped me navigate the once foreign world of agents, publishers, and authors. Thank you for all your help and for being both a loving mother and a mentor. I love you, Mom. I miss you so very much.

A special thanks goes to Jody Berman for her invaluable assistance in the initial preparation of this manuscript. Her expert editing skills helped me take my ideas and transform them into a real book. Thank you, Jody.

My gratitude is deeply extended to all the friends and family who supported me in what was such a huge undertaking. I would especially like to acknowledge the kindness and encouragement of Dr. Jacky Pepper, Eric Wolfe, and my longtime friend Abbé Sloven. Wholehearted thanks to Dr. Gil Gutierrez, a family physician and personal friend, for his patient referrals, and thank you to P. J. Stawicki and Debbie Wolff, excellent personal trainers who were kind enough to refer their clients to me. To my in-laws, Edna and Harry Brill, who have since passed on. You were warm and loving people who were so good to me.

To the esteemed Dr. Jennifer Mieres, thank you kindly for your informative foreword. I am honored that you agreed to contribute to my book.

Also, many thanks to my patients for their willingness to try out my plan and for helping me bring it to the public. I wish you all continued success in following the program, keeping your cholesterol down, and remaining in good health.

Thank you to my original editor, Lindsay Orman, for the countless hours you spent poring over my manuscript, culling out the extraneous matter, and making it succinct and reader-friendly. Your editing expertise truly amazes me, and I greatly appreciate your talents.

Finally, I would like to acknowledge Elysia Liang, my new editor, for this revision at Penguin Random House. Your invitation to revise this book is much appreciated as well as all your invaluable help in reviewing the new manuscript.

Index

About the Author

Janet Bond Brill, PhD, RDN, FAND, was born and raised in New York City, the daughter of a prominent stage and screen actor and a psychoanalyst. At the age of sixteen, she graduated from Walden School in Manhattan and enrolled at the University of Miami, earning her BS in biology. Taking a break from academia, she worked as a flight attendant for Pan American World Airways for seven years.

Returning to South Florida, she earned both her doctoral degree and master's degree in exercise physiology from the University of Miami, in addition to a second master's degree in nutrition science from Florida International University, graduating both universities with academic honors.

Dr. Brill has been a nutritionist in private practice for many years, specializing in cardiovascular disease prevention. Dr. Brill is a registered and licensed dietitian and nutritionist, certified personal trainer, wellness coach, and former adjunct faculty member at the University of Miami, where she taught both graduate and undergraduate classes in exercise physiology, sports nutrition, and wellness. Her research on the cholesterol-lowering effects of her healthy lifestyle program has been published in the *International Journal of Obesity.* She has also published scientific research in the *International Journal of Sport Nutrition* as well as articles on health and fitness for the popular press.

Dr. Brill currently resides in Pennsylvania and South Florida and enjoys an active lifestyle, practicing what she preaches, having completed four marathons and countless 5k, 10k, and half-marathon road races. She enjoys spending free time with her husband, three children, two grandchildren, and three dogs, Lilly, River, and Maggie.

Also available from

JANET BOND BRILL, PhD, RDN, FAND

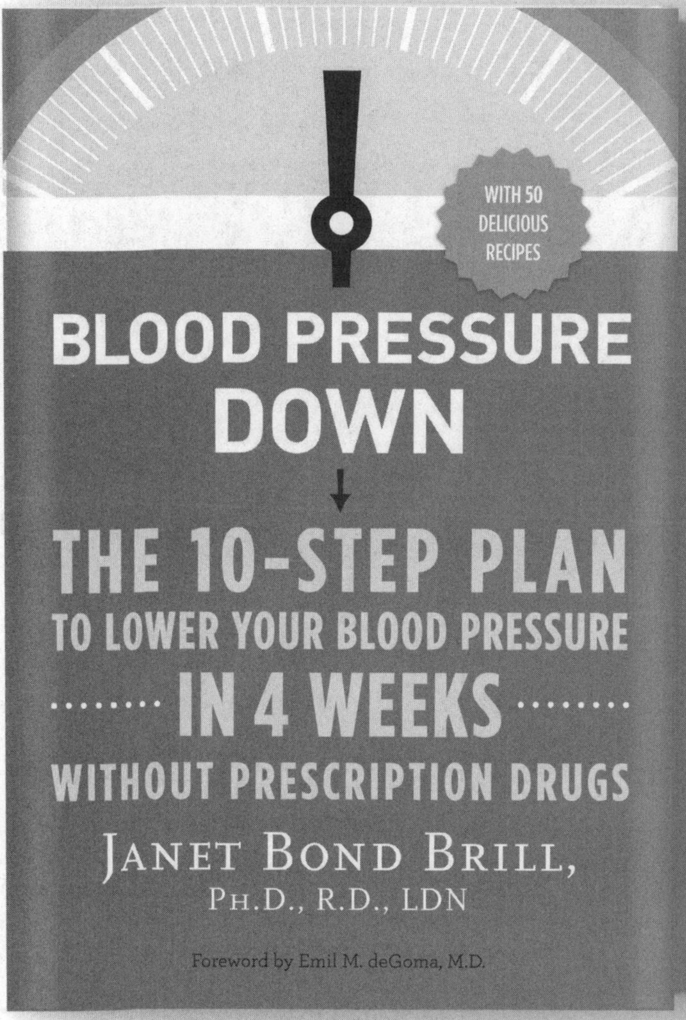

WITH 50 DELICIOUS RECIPES

BLOOD PRESSURE DOWN

THE 10-STEP PLAN TO LOWER YOUR BLOOD PRESSURE IN 4 WEEKS WITHOUT PRESCRIPTION DRUGS

JANET BOND BRILL, PH.D., R.D., LDN

Foreword by Emil M. deGoma, M.D.

HARMONY

Available now wherever books are sold